The Diabetic Dessert Cookbook

The Diabetic Dessert Cookbook

COLEEN HOWARD

Foreword by **GEORGE SEBERG, M. D.**

AVON BOOKS NEW YORK

The recipes herein are not meant to replace the advice of a licensed health care practitioner. The reader should consult his or her own physician regarding any dietary requirements or restrictions.

The nutritional values were provided by computer software from ESHA Research, Salem, Oregon. Isomalt® is a registered trademark, distrubuted in the United States by Palatini, Inc., U.S.A.

AVON BOOKS
A division of
The Hearst Corporation
1350 Avenue of the Americas
New York, New York 10019

Copyright © 1997 by Coleen Howard
Cover illustration by Gary Head
Published by arrangement with the author
Visit our website at http://www.AvonBooks.com
ISBN: 0-380-78823-3

Library of Congress Cataloging in Publication Data:

Howard, Coleen.
    The diabetic dessert cookbook / Coleen Howard ; foreword by George Seberg.
        p.   cm.
    Includes index.
    1. Diabetes—Diet therapy—Recipes.   2. Desserts.   I. Title.
    RC662.H69   1997   96-36961
    641.8'6—dc21   CIP

First Avon Books Trade Printing: April 1997

AVON TRADEMARK REG. U.S. PAT. OFF. AND IN OTHER COUNTRIES, MARCA REGISTRADA, HECHO EN U.S.A.

QPM   10   9   8   7   6   5   4   3   2

This book is dedicated to my husband, Charles, who has provided the inspiration for this book and supported all my efforts in life. Because of his love and his encouragement, it is possible to share this book with you.

He deserves all the sweetness of life itself.

About the Author

Coleen Howard is a nutrition consultant who has been making and writing about candy for years. Several of her cookbooks have already been published. She lectures and teaches on current nutritional guidelines and changes in the health care field related to diabetes and other sugar diseases. She also appears on television cooking shows and radio talk shows.

Coleen was inspired to make desserts without sugar because her husband is diabetic. With the need of proper diet for diabetics in mind, she created these dessert recipes.

Millions of people are afflicted with diabetes and other diseases that require special diets. Many of these diets restrict sugar and fat altogether, or require that only small amounts be ingested. Guidelines for persons afflicted with sugar-related diseases have changed. Today, diets include natural sugars (fructose) and some polyunsaturated fats, important to a healthy, stable individual.

Desserts can be made without sugar and with healthy ingredients. The author's inspiration to produce good and fun foods for her husband brought about the creation of these desserts to be shared by all.

Through the author's knowledge and experiments, as well as her husband's willingness to taste it all, the following no- and low-sugar desserts were developed. Now all can enjoy and reap the benefits of these efforts—her recipes and his taste buds!

Foreword

As a practicing internist for the last twenty years, it has been a constant battle to find appropriate diets for treatment of the major medical maladies of our time. Diet plays a pivotal role in diabetes, heart disease, cancer and most other chronic medical problems. The medical literature is replete with different dietary regimes for every possible medical illness. The lay literature has comparable amounts of data about everything from pineapple diets to Weight Watchers. The failure or success of many diets rests upon the dedication of the dieter and the type of foods that he or she is able to ingest without exceeding certain caloric limits.

I feel that the acceptable and effective diets available in our country today have a common thread running through them. The best characteristics of all diets contain elements that are essential for weight loss in an obese individual, control of the blood sugar in a diabetic, or control of the lipids in severe hyperlipidemia. I think that a strong but neglected part of all diets is the exercise component. If a person does not change the activity level at the same time they change their intake levels, there can be no weight loss.

The common elements in all diets are what you eat, when you eat, and how you eat it. How you eat is particularly important. Sit down at a specific time. The food should be served in a reasonable manner. The amounts of food should be carefully controlled. The patient should not have the distraction of extra portions or prohibited food being readily available. It is important to make sure that the meal setting is quiet and stress-free. It should occur at the same time every day. It takes a minimum of twenty minutes to eat. It also takes twenty minutes for the brain to get the signal from the stomach that it is full. If you clock the average eating time in a busy restaurant with a stopwatch, you will find that five minutes is more the norm than twenty minutes.

But what you eat is the key in any diet. A balance must be maintained between fats, carbohydrates and proteins. Fat should constitute less than thirty percent of the diet, and carbohydrates should be high and protein low. With that in mind, it is important to modify the composition of the foods that one eats in each disease state and avoid certain types and quantities of foods. Unfortunately in America today, too many people eat fast food and other calorically empty foods that mightily contribute to a high instance of heart disease, diabetes, obesity and ongoing chronic medical problems. It is very important to make a strategic shift in the types of food products that we consume. However, I strongly feel that shifts in the diet must be made gradually by substitutions, exchanges and cross-referencing one type of food for another. These changes can be made using the available products that we have today. With minimal effort, most people can come up with a program to place themselves in a healthier eating bracket than they have previously maintained.

I am delighted to introduce a book that goes a long way to help diabetics make the transition to safe eating. With her *Diabetic Dessert Cookbook,* Mrs. Howard adds another arrow to our armament to fight off ''bad eating.'' She takes out the simple sugars, the chemicals and the calorie-adding techniques from dessert making. She gives us an alternate choice in our diets for the psychological sweet tooth, which we all have trouble denying. She has time and taste tested each one of the recipes. I wholeheartedly endorse her efforts. With this book comes a large step in the move toward better eating for the health-conscious and for people who are on restricted diets for a multitude of medical illnesses.

George Seberg, M.D., Internist

Contents

The Diabetic Dessert Cookbook

Introduction

Over a century ago the first case of diabetes mellitus was diagnosed. Thus began the search for the treatment, cure and management of this debilitating and life-threatening disease. The value of research has been demonstrated by the resulting constant change in diabetes management through the years. It is now possible for the diabetic to remain active and have a full, productive and long life.

Research has defined two types of diabetes, Type I and Type II. Type I requires insulin and Type II requires oral medication. In addition to medication, a program of exercise, weight control and nutrition is significant in improvement of the overall health of the diabetic.

The goal for the prevention and treatment of the acute complications of diabetes mellitus, such as hypoglycemia, short-term illnesses and exercise-related problems, renal disease, autonomic neuropathy, hypertension and cardiovascular disease, has led us to current diabetic management programs.

Many changes supporting and enhancing the quality of life have occurred through the years. Major breakthroughs in nutrition have provided less rigid diets and more options in those diets. For instance, in 1921 the diabetic was allowed ten percent protein in the daily diet. Later research raised the daily allowance to ten to twenty percent. The diet for the diabetic in 1921 was rigid. In today's world, the diabetic works on an individual basis with health care providers to use improved dietary supplements to better enjoy meals as well as provide the body with the proper nutrition.

Through research, and with today's standards, it has been found that not only does sugar play an integral part in daily nutrition, but fat content is important as well. Today there are polyunsaturated fats, and sugar and salt substitutes that allow a higher quality serving and more foods for consumption within the dietary needs of the individual. Current nutritional standards even include higher daily percentages of fructose and carbohydrate consumption. The current guidelines health care professionals follow as well as those listed by the American Diabetic Association set nutritional values on a daily basis, including calories, carbohydrates, cholesterol, fat, fiber and protein. These values are also used in the daily nutrition of the individual diabetic.

While all of us need to be aware of nutritional values, this information is of particular importance to those with diabetes, cardiovascular disease, and other sugar-related disease. Today, people are increasingly aware of food consumption and the need for good daily nutrition. The best preventative medicine we have is controlling what we eat. These recipes are to make nutritional planning more interesting and satisfying, but are not "in addition" to current food intake.

The most recent research recognizes the need for daily food consumption to be enjoyable. This is especially true for a person who feels deprived and craves certain nutrients such as sugar. For the diabetic, there is a craving for sugar. It is important for the diabetic and those with other sugar-related diseases to satisfy these cravings.

There are over three million people in the United States alone diagnosed with diabetes mellitus and many more not yet diagnosed. This does not include those with related medical complications of heart disease and hypoglycemia. My husband is one of the three million with diabetes mellitus; through him I learned about the cravings and the need to satisfy those cravings. Thus began my quest for good nutrition and enjoyment of food on a daily basis, and the result is this book.

This cookbook is for all who desire good nutrition and want to enjoy sweet treats. These dessert recipes were developed over a long period of time. They are original recipes. Each recipe has been designed with nutritional values in mind, as well as providing the sweets that we all desire and sometimes crave.

The recipes use ingredients that are friendly to the human body, including polyunsaturated fats, sugar substitutes, fresh fruits, vegetables and carob. Many of the recipes contain zero fat and zero sugar. Each recipe contains the measurement of the five main categories of nutritional values per serving. In the appendix you will find a complete analysis of each recipe.

My goal with this dessert cookbook is to provide everyone with sweet treats that will not harm the human body and will provide enjoyment for the millions of people with sugar-related disease, cardiovascular disease, those with medical problems who feel deprived of their treats and for those who are strong and healthy and wish to remain so through good nutrition without deprivation of food.

May you enjoy these easy-to-make dessert recipes that feed the body and the soul with the sweetness of life itself.

Coleen Howard

Candies, Squares, and Dessert Bars

Candy-Making Tips

All recipes in this book are original recipes by Coleen Howard. Each recipe has been tested to perfection.

ARTIFICIAL SWEETENER: Artificial sweetener used in these recipes is in liquid form. Granulated artificial sweeteners are acceptable. Use the same amount as noted for the liquid form. It is advisable to use granulated artificial sweeteners when used as a coating for the finished product.

CAROB: Carob is the replacement for chocolate. Melt carob as you would chocolate. Use your double boiler with hot, not boiling, water. If you do not have a double boiler, a metal bowl placed over a bowl of hot water will suffice. When carob is melted, it may form a soft ball. Cool to the point of handling the carob. Then knead in the remaining ingredients. This will not change the texture of your finished product. When the carob has melted, add the artificial sweetener. Your desserts, including truffles, will have the flavor of chocolate. If you prefer a more liquid form of melted carob, add polyunsaturated oil (one tablespoon per cup of melted carob). Add until desired liquidity is reached. Remember to change the nutritional values to include the additional oil.

You can purchase a presweetened carob. If you prefer to use presweetened carob, note any change in nutritional values. Most presweetened carob uses non-nutritional sweeteners. The recipes in this book use unsweetened carob.

COOKING STAGES: If you use a candy thermometer, cook your candy as follows:

Cold Water Stage	Equivalent Candy Thermometer Temperature
"Soft ball"	234–240°
"Hard ball"	250–269°
"Crack" or "Soft crack"	270–290°
"Hard crack" or "Brittle"	300–310°

When using a candy thermometer, cook your candy to the exact temperature as noted above. If you are cooking in altitudes over 3,000 feet (especially for creamy candies), subtract two to four degrees.

If you are using the cold water method for testing candy, drop ½ teaspoon of the cooking candy mixture into one cup of cold water. Be sure water is very cold. Let stand for approximately one minute and then check the firmness of the cooled candy with your fingers.

DIETETIC: This refers to items that can be purchased in the grocery store in the diet section. These items include canned fruits and vegetables packed in water rather than heavy sugary syrups. If you cannot find these items, then purchase the regular fruits and place them in a colander. Run cold water over the fruit to remove the sugary syrup.

EXTRACTS: Do not use artificial extracts in these recipes. They may prevent the candy from setting properly and may also alter the taste.

FRUIT: The fruits noted in the recipes are fresh fruit unless specified as dried fruit.

GRAININESS: Once a spoon is used to mix and dissolve the candy, rinse the spoon and dry. Do this often to remove any granules. Do not scrape your cooking pot. The grains will adhere to the sides of the pot. Leave them in the pot—not in your candy!

GRANOLA: Check the nutritional values on the package of granola. Some granola contains sugar. The granola in these recipes does not contain sugar.

INGREDIENTS: The ingredients for the recipes in this book are readily available in your local grocery stores and health food stores. Isomalt® (sugar substitute and hardening agent) is listed below for purchase by mail. Wherever possible, ingredients that do not contain sugar are used.

ISOMALT®: Isomalt® is a sugar substitute for specific recipes. It is a hardening agent. The remaining recipes use any liquid or granulated non-nutritional sweeteners on the market.

To make powdered Isomalt®, place the Isomalt® in a blender. Blend on highest speed until Isomalt® becomes a powder. Store in an airtight container. Use the powdered Isomalt® in all recipes calling for "powdered Isomalt®." Use Isomalt® in its original form in all other recipes.

Isomalt® may be purchased from Palatini, Inc. U.S.A., c/o Material Trans Action, Inc., 2741 N. Foundation Drive, South Bend, Indiana 46634. At the time of this publication the product was not available in retail stores.

MAPLE SYRUP: Some recipes call for "sugarless maple syrup." Check the labels carefully when purchasing sugarless maple syrup. Maple syrup is a sugar unto itself.

MARGARINE: The margarine used in these recipes is unsalted. Where salt is indicated in a recipe, a salt substitute may be used.

MEASUREMENTS: Carob is measured by placing small pieces (about the size of chocolate chips) in the measuring cup. This is for all carob (for chocolate flavor) recipes. Other items such as shredded coconut and nuts are all measured as the recipe indicates. The shredded coconut is measured after shredding a whole coconut or purchasing coconut that is already shredded. Measure chopped nuts and fruits after the chopping process.

¼ teaspoon	=	1 milliliter
½ teaspoon	=	2 milliliters
1 teaspoon	=	5 milliliters
2 teaspoons	=	10 milliliters
½ ounce	=	1 tablespoon, or 3 teaspoons, or 15 milliliters
1 ounce	=	2 tablespoons, or 6 teaspoons, or 30 milliliters
8 ounces	=	1 cup, or 16 tablespoons, or 48 teaspoons or 250 milliliters
2.2 pounds	=	1 kilogram

MOLDS: Candy molds may be used in place of pans or cookie sheets. There are many interesting and fun shapes available. You may also use candy cutters and cookie cutters for other interesting shapes.

NUTS: The nuts used in these recipes are unsalted unless salted nuts are specified.

OTHER INGREDIENTS: The items used here are no-sugar and no-salt ingredients. Use dietetic peanut butter, margarine and other ingredients. This will assure the correct nutritional value per recipe.

PAN SIZE: Use the pan size noted in each recipe. This will give you the accurate depth of the dessert for proper nutritional values.

PER SERVING SIZE: All recipes in this book are based on a per serving size of one inch by one inch squares. The depth per square is ½ to ¾ inch.

STORAGE: All desserts should be kept in a cool, dry place. The recipes in this book can be frozen for six months.

TEXTURE: The area in which you live may affect the texture of your desserts. For instance, hard candies may become sticky if you live in a hot, humid climate. The candies should all be treated as any candy made with sugar.

UTENSILS: Use nonstick pans or cookie sheets to place the cooked candy for cooling. This eliminates the use of oil. If you are using candy molds that require the use of oil, use a diabetic spray instead.

When cooking your ingredients, do NOT use a nonstick pot. When candy is poured into a pan or mold, the extra granules will stick to the pot. You do not want those granules in your completed dessert.

Citrus Candy

2 cups orange, lemon, lime or grapefruit rind, cut
   in 1" square pieces
6 cups cold water
1/8 teaspoon artificial sweetener
1 cup powdered Isomalt®

Wash the rind well. Cut away white inner skin from rind. Cut rind in 1" squares. Put rind, water and sweetener in a 2-quart saucepan. Bring to a boil. Cook until water and sugar substitute are completely absorbed by rind. Once absorbed, remove from pan and place the cooked rind on waxed paper to cool and dry. When cool enough to handle, roll pieces in powdered Isomalt®. Return coated pieces to waxed paper. Let the rind dry for approximately 24 hours. Wrap individual pieces in plastic wrap. Store in refrigerator or freezer. Yield: 24 pieces. Size: 1" square x 1/2" deep per piece.

Nutritional Values (per piece)

Calories:	3.33	Fiber:	.136 g
Carbohydrates:	1 g	Protein:	.061 g
Cholesterol:	0 mg	Sodium:	.12 mg
Fat:	.008 g		

◎

Coated Citrus Candy

2 cups orange, lemon, lime or grapefruit rind, cut
   in 1" square pieces
6 cups cold water
⅛ teaspoon artificial sweetener
2 cups carob

Wash the rind well. Cut away white inner skin from rind. Cut rind
in 1" squares. Put rind, water and sugar substitute in a 2-quart saucepan. Bring to a boil. Cook until water and sugar substitute completely
absorbed by rind. Once absorbed, remove from pan and place the
cooked rind on waxed paper to cool and dry. Let the rind dry for
approximately 24 hours. Melt carob and sweetener in double boiler.
Dip citrus candy in melted carob. Place on waxed paper to set. Yield:
60 pieces. Size 1" square x ⅛" deep per piece.

Nutritional Values (per piece)

Calories:	19.2	Fiber	.054 g
Carbohydrates:	2.47 g	Protein	.586 g
Cholesterol:	.302 mg	Sodium:	.048 mg
Fat:	.835 g		

⊚

Yummy Bananas

4 cups carob
⅛ teaspoon artificial sweetener
1 cup dried, crumbled bananas

Melt carob and artificial sweetener in double boiler. Crumble dried bananas by placing bananas between two pieces of waxed paper. Using a rolling pin, roll over bananas to crumble. Add crumbled bananas to carob. Mix well. Place in a 9" x 9" square pan. Cool. Cut into 1" squares, ¾" deep. Yield: 85 pieces.

Nutritional Values (per piece)

Calories:	54.6	Fiber:	.09 g
Carbohydrates:	6.89 g	Protein:	1.63 g
Cholesterol:	.854 mg	Sodium:	.035 mg
Fat:	2.37 g		

9

Truffles

4 cups carob
⅛ teaspoon artificial sweetener
1 teaspoon powdered instant coffee
1 cup finely chopped peanuts

Melt carob in double boiler. Add artificial sweetener to melted carob and stir well. You may use molds for fancy-shaped truffles or place mixture in a bowl to cool. When cool enough to form a ball, form into 1" diameter balls and roll in either instant coffee or chopped peanuts (not both). Place on waxed paper. Place truffles in refrigerator for 20 minutes to set. Yield: 90 pieces.

Nutritional Values (per piece)

Calories:	57.2		Fiber:	.112 g
Carbohydrates:	5.88 g		Protein:	1.88 g
Cholesterol:	.806 mg		Sodium:	.097 mg
Fat:	3.02 g			

Coconut Delight

3 cups shredded coconut
3 large egg whites, lightly beaten
2 teaspoons rum extract
4 cups carob
⅛ teaspoon artificial sweetener

Mix 2 cups coconut and lightly beaten egg whites. Add rum extract. Shape into 1" diameter balls. Place on cookie sheet. Preheat oven to 350° F. Bake for 20 to 25 minutes. Coconut balls will be lightly brown. While the coconut balls are still warm, reshape any balls that may have lost their round shape during baking. Cool the coconut balls. Melt carob with artificial sweetener in double boiler. Dip coconut balls in carob. Place on waxed paper to cool. When cool enough to handle, roll in remaining coconut. Place in refrigerator to set. Yield: 75 pieces.

Nutritional Values (per piece)

Calories:	22.4		Fiber:	.301 g
Carbohydrates:	1.74 g		Protein:	.523 g
Cholesterol:	.181 mg		Sodium:	1.88 mg
Fat:	1.57 g			

◉

Coconut Drops

1 cup light Philadelphia cream cheese
2 cups shredded coconut

Mix cream cheese and coconut. Drop by 1" diameter spoonfuls onto waxed paper. Refrigerate. Yield: 90 pieces.

- *For a festive touch, color the coconut with food coloring before you mix with the cream cheese. Place in small paper cups in a gift box of sugarless candies for someone you love.*

Nutritional Values (per piece)

Calories:	19.2		Fiber:	.271 g
Carbohydrates:	.509 g		Protein:	.291 g
Cholesterol:	2.83 mg		Sodium:	8.21 mg
Fat:	1.87 g			

Creamy Strawberries

4 cups carob
⅛ teaspoon artificial sweetener
12 ounces light Philadelphia cream cheese
2 cups crushed strawberries, fresh or frozen

Melt carob and artificial sweetener in double boiler. Mix cream cheese and strawberries. Add to melted carob. Mix well. Pour into a 9" x 9" square pan. Let cool and set in refrigerator for at least 2 hours. Cut into 1" squares, ½" deep. Place in small paper cups. Yield: 80 pieces.

Nutritional Values (per piece)

Calories:	58.7	Fiber:	.064 g
Carbohydrates:	6.66 g	Protein:	2.31 g
Cholesterol:	1.66 mg	Sodium:	25.5 mg
Fat:	2.51 g		

Fruit Surprise

½ cup whipping cream
1 cup finely chopped carob
2 tablespoons rum extract
½ cup shredded coconut
½ cup chopped almonds
¼ cup chopped dried banana chips
¼ cup chopped dried pineapple

Scald the cream in a 2-quart saucepan. Remove from heat. Add chopped carob. Stir until smooth. Return to heat. Let cook for 5 to 10 minutes. Add rum extract, coconut, almonds, banana chips and pineapple chips. Pour into an 8" x 8" square pan. Refrigerate 6 hours before cutting. Remove from refrigerator and cut into 1" squares. Shape each square into balls 1" in diameter. Place the balls on a plate and refrigerate for 4 hours to allow candy to set. Yield: 80 pieces.

Nutritional Values (per piece)

Calories:	26.2		Fiber:	.148 g
Carbohydrates:	2.11 mg		Protein:	.643 g
Cholesterol:	2.26 mg		Sodium:	.758 mg
Fat:	1.77 g			

Rascal Raspberries

2 cups whole raspberries
4 cups carob
⅛ teaspoon artificial sweetener
1 teaspoon vanilla extract

Wash and drain raspberries. Place raspberries in a 9" x 9" square pan lined with waxed paper. Melt carob and artificial sweetener in double boiler. Add vanilla extract. Pour mixture over raspberries. Let cool and cut into 1" squares, ½" deep. Yield: 90 pieces.

Nutritional Values (per piece)

Calories:	49.2		Fiber:	.108 g
Carbohydrates:	5.85 g		Protein:	1.52 g
Cholesterol:	.806 mg		Sodium:	.001 mg
Fat:	2.23 g			

Crunch Bars

1 cup carob
1/8 teaspoon artificial sweetener
2 tablespoons vegetable shortening
1 1/2 cups coarsely crumbled saltine crackers

Melt the carob, artificial sweetener and vegetable shortening in a double boiler. Stir until smooth. Add the crumbled saltine crackers. Place in a loaf pan. Press firmly. Cool. Cut into 1/4" x 1" bars, 1/2" deep. Yield: 36 pieces.

Nutritional Values (per piece)

Calories:	80.1		Fiber:	.128 g
Carbohydrates:	10.3 g		Protein:	2.31 g
Cholesterol:	1.01 mg		Sodium:	30.1 mg
Fat:	3.33 g			

Happy Trails

4 cups carob
3 cups dry granola
3 cups dry rice cereal
1 cup chopped peanuts
1 teaspoon vanilla extract

Melt carob in double boiler. Set aside. Mix together the granola, rice and peanuts. Add to melted carob. Stir. Add vanilla extract and stir. Spread mixture evenly on a cookie sheet lined with waxed paper. Press lightly. Cool and cut into 1" squares, ½" deep. Yield: 85 pieces.

Nutritional Values (per piece)

Calories:	85.6		Fiber:	.582 g
Carbohydrates:	9.48 g		Protein:	2.59 g
Cholesterol:	.854 mg		Sodium:	7.81 mg
Fat:	4.38 g			

෧

Raisin Clusters

1 cup carob
⅛ teaspoon artificial sweetener
½ cup raisins

Melt carob and artificial sweetener in double boiler. Remove from
heat. Stir in raisins. Place by 1" diameter × ½" deep spoonfuls on
waxed paper to cool. Yield: 36 pieces.

Nutritional Values (per piece)

Calories:	35.9	Fiber:	.07 g
Carbohydrates:	5.05 g	Protein:	1 g
Cholesterol:	.504 mg	Sodium:	.242 mg
Fat:	1.4 g		

☺

Peanut Butter and
Cream Cheese Kisses

½ *pound carob*
⅛ *teaspoon artificial sweetener*
12 ounces Philadelphia light cream cheese
1 cup crunchy dietetic peanut butter

Melt carob and artificial sweetener in double boiler. Mix together cream cheese and peanut butter. Roll mixture into 1" diameter balls. Dip in melted carob. Place on waxed paper to set. Stores well in refrigerator or freezer. Yield: 80 pieces.

Nutritional Values (per piece)

Calories:	36		Fiber:	.212 g
Carbohydrates:	2.4 g		Protein:	1.79 g
Cholesterol:	.975 mg		Sodium:	26 mg
Fat:	2.21 g			

Peanut Butter Cups

4 cups carob
⅛ teaspoon artificial sweetener
2 cups smooth dietetic peanut butter

Melt carob and artificial sweetener in double boiler. Remove from heat. Pour melted carob into chocolate molds. Fill to half full. Then add peanut butter, leaving enough room at the top to add more carob. Add enough carob to completely cover. Refrigerate until set, approximately 20 minutes. Cut into 1" square x ½" deep. Yield: 80 pieces.

Nutritional Values (per piece)

Calories:	91.9		Fiber:	.422 g
Carbohydrates:	7.25 g		Protein:	3.42 g
Cholesterol:	.907 mg		Sodium:	1.09 mg
Fat:	5.85 g			

Peanut Butter-Potato Pinwheels

*½ cup cold mashed potatoes (no milk or seasoning
   added)*
⅛ teaspoon salt or salt substitute
4 cups powdered Isomalt®
½ teaspoon vanilla extract
1 cup dietetic peanut butter

To potatoes, add salt or salt substitute and 1 cup powdered Isomalt®.
Beat well. Add vanilla and turn half of mixture onto board that has
been lightly dusted with powdered Isomalt®. Roll into a rectangle
¼" thick. Spread with half the peanut butter. Roll up from short
side, jelly roll fashion, to 1" diameter. Repeat with remaining mixture. Chill for at least 2 hours. Slice ¼" thick. Yield: 75 pieces.

Nutritional Values (per piece)

Calories:	21.7	Fiber:	.25 g
Carbohydrates:	1.1 g	Protein:	.85 g
Cholesterol:	0 mg	Sodium:	.671 mg
Fat:	1.7 g		

Chocolate Peanut Butter Fudge

2 cups finely chopped carob
⅛ teaspoon artificial sweetener
⅔ cup cold mashed potatoes (no milk or seasoning added)
½ cup dietetic peanut butter (crunchy works best)
⅛ teaspoon salt substitute

Melt carob and artificial sweetener in double boiler. Set aside. Mix together mashed potatoes, peanut butter and salt substitute. Add mixture to melted carob. Pour into a 9" x 9" square pan. Spread evenly. Cool until set. Cut into 1" squares, ½" deep. Yield: 90 pieces.

Nutritional Values (per piece)

Calories:	33.5	Fiber:	.114 g
Carbohydrates:	3.37 g	Protein:	1.12 g
Cholesterol:	.403 mg	Sodium:	.317 mg
Fat:	1.82 g		

Peanut Butter and Banana Fudge

⅔ cup cold mashed potatoes (no milk or seasoning
  added)
⅛ teaspoon salt substitute
⅓ cup dietetic peanut butter (crunchy works best)
¼ cup mashed, ripe bananas

Mix together the mashed potatoes and salt substitute. Add peanut
butter and bananas. Press mixture into an 8" x 8" square pan. Refrigerate until set, approximately 4 hours. Cut into 1" squares, ½" deep.
This is a soft fudge and so yummy. Yield: 48 pieces.

Nutritional Values (per piece)

Calories:	14.2	Fiber:	.18 g
Carbohydrates:	1.15 g	Protein:	.545 g
Cholesterol:	0 mg	Sodium:	.462 mg
Fat:	.942 g		

Peanut Butter Balls

3 cups shredded coconut
½ cup dietetic peanut butter (smooth or crunchy)
1 teaspoon vanilla extract
2 cups shredded coconut

Combine 3 cups coconut with peanut butter and vanilla extract. Mix well. Shape into 1" diameter balls. Roll balls in the 2 cups shredded coconut. Coat thoroughly. Place in pan lined with waxed paper. Chill thoroughly. Yield: 80 pieces.

Nutritional Values (per piece)

Calories:	16.4		Fiber:	.294 g
Carbohydrates:	.649 g		Protein:	.451 g
Cholesterol:	0 mg		Sodium:	.496 mg
Fat:	1.47 g			

Peanut Butter Bars

¹/₄ cup margarine
¹/₂ teaspoon sugar substitute
2 eggs
rind of ¹/₂ lemon, grated
2 cups sifted all-purpose flour
1¹/₂ teaspoons cinnamon
1 8-ounce can salted peanuts

Cream margarine. Add sugar substitute, eggs and lemon rind. Mix well. Add flour and cinnamon. Mix well. Add peanuts and stir. Shape into bars 1" x 1¹/₂" x 1" thick. Pat firmly. Cover with waxed paper and allow to dry overnight.

Heat oven to 375° F. Bake the bars 12 to 15 minutes. Let cool. Yield: 36 pieces.

• *For an additional treat, dip bars in melted carob.*

Nutritional Values (per piece)

Calories:	77.5		Fiber:	.663 g
Carbohydrates:	6.7 g		Protein:	2.56 g
Cholesterol:	11.8 g		Sodium:	4.05 mg
Fat:	4.75 g			

Peanut Butter Fudge

²/₃ cup cold mashed potatoes (no milk or seasoning added)
½ cup crunchy dietetic peanut butter
⅛ cup salt or salt substitute
4 cups powdered Isomalt®

Grease an 8" x 8" pan. Mix potatoes with peanut butter and salt. Gradually stir in Isomalt®, mixing well. Press into greased pan. Let stand until firm. Then cut into 1" squares, ½" deep. See if anyone can guess you used potatoes! (No instant potatoes please. I tried it, it doesn't work). Yield: 80 pieces.

Nutritional Values (per piece)

Calories:	10.9	Fiber:	.129 g
Carbohydrates:	.698 g	Protein:	.414 g
Cholesterol:	0 mg	Sodium:	.185 mg
Fat:	.797 g		

☺

Friendly Dates

¾ cup finely chopped dried figs
¾ cup finely chopped dried dates
¾ cup finely chopped English walnuts
2 tablespoons grated orange rind
2 tablespoons lemon juice
60 English walnut halves

If the figs and dates are too dry, place in a bowl of hot water to moisten. Place the figs, dates and chopped walnuts in a blender. Blend well. Place mixture on a pastry board. Sprinkle with the grated orange rind and lemon juice. Knead thoroughly until well blended. Form the mixture in a long, sausage-shaped roll, 1" in diameter. Cut the roll into ¾" thick slices. Place on waxed paper. Put 1 walnut half on top of each piece of candy. Press into candy. Allow candy to dry and become firm. Store in a cool place. May be frozen. Yield: 60 pieces.

Nutritional Values (per piece)

Calories:	57.8		Fiber:	.785 g
Carbohydrates:	5.24 g		Protein:	1.09 g
Cholesterol:	0 mg		Sodium:	1.07 mg
Fat:	4.14 g			

Candied Nuts

3 cups sugar-free maple syrup
½ cup Isomalt®
½ cup water
4 cups English walnuts or pecan halves

Put maple syrup, Isomalt® and water in a heavy saucepan. Bring to a boil and let the mixture cook down to approximately 2 cups or until it reaches a hard crack stage. Add nuts and coat thoroughly. Pour nuts onto a cookie sheet. Separate nuts and allow to cool and dry. Break or cut into 1" squares, ¼" deep. Yield: 90 pieces.

Nutritional Values (per piece)

Calories:	40.9		Fiber:	.201 g
Carbohydrates:	4.17 g		Protein:	.636 g
Cholesterol:	0 mg		Sodium:	15.6 mg
Fat:	2.75 g			

Granola Delight

4 tablespoons margarine
4 tablespoons sugar-free maple syrup
1 cup finely chopped dates
1 cup granola
1 cup shredded coconut

Place the margarine and maple syrup in a heavy, 2-quart saucepan. Cook over low heat until margarine is melted and blended into the maple syrup. Add the chopped dates. Continue cooking and stir constantly until the dates are almost dissolved. Remove from heat. Stir in granola. Allow to cool. When cool enough to handle, roll into balls of 1" diameter and immediately roll the ball in the shredded coconut. Yield: 60 pieces.

Nutritional Values (per piece)

Calories:	31.3		Fiber:	.562 g
Carbohydrates:	3.97 g		Protein:	.358 g
Cholesterol:	0 mg		Sodium:	4.05 mg
Fat:	1.77 g			

Stuffed Dates

48 pitted dried dates
¹/₄ cup dietetic peanut butter
¹/₂ cup chopped pecans

Place the dried dates in hot water. Set aside until dates are soft. Mix the peanut butter with the chopped pecans. Fill each date with 1 teaspoon of the peanut butter and pecan mixture. Refigerate. Yield: 48 pieces.

• *Put shredded coconut on top of stuffed date. Not only is it pretty but it tastes good, too!*

Nutritional Values (per piece)			
Calories:	42	Fiber:	.855 g
Carbohydrates:	7.46 g	Protein:	.603 g
Cholesterol:	0 mg	Sodium:	.376 mg
Fat:	1.54 g		

Sweet Almonds

2 cups almonds
¼ cup margarine
⅛ teaspoon artificial sweetener

Blanch almonds by dropping into boiling water for 3 to 4 minutes. Remove and drain. Remove skin from almonds. Place the margarine in a heavy iron skillet. Cook over medium heat. When margarine is melted, add the blanched almonds. Cook until the almonds are golden brown. Remove from heat. Place the almonds in a grinder or blender. Grind or blend until mixture forms a paste. Add artificial sweetener and blend. Form into 1" diameter balls. Place on waxed paper. Flatten with a spatula. Allow to cool to room temperature. Refrigerate. Yield: 80 pieces.

Nutritional Values (per piece)

Calories:	26.3	Fiber:	.353 g
Carbohydrates:	.674 g	Protein:	.744 g
Cholesterol:	0 mg	Sodium:	.378 mg
Fat:	2.47 g		

☺

Dream Balls

1 large, ripe banana
½ pound pitted, finely chopped dates
1 cup finely chopped English walnuts
2 cups shredded coconut

Mash the banana thoroughly with a fork. Add the chopped dates.
Mix thoroughly. Add the chopped English walnuts. Mix thoroughly.
Form into 1" diameter balls and roll in shredded coconut. Be sure
to coat thoroughly. Refrigerate 4 hours uncovered. Yield: 60 pieces.

Nutritional Values (per piece)

Calories:	25		Fiber:	.414 g
Carbohydrates:	3.59 g		Protein:	.381 g
Cholesterol:	0 mg		Sodium:	.332 mg
Fat:	1.26 g			

＠

Sweet Sesame

1 cup sesame seeds
⅛ teaspoon artificial sweetener
¼ teaspoon almond extract
½ cup raisins
20 English walnut halves

Place the sesame seeds in a blender. Blend until smooth. Turn onto a cutting board and knead in the artificial sweetener. Knead in the almond extract. Add the raisins and knead thoroughly. Pinch off small amounts and shape into 1" diameter balls. Place on waxed paper. Flatten the balls with a spatula. Place an English walnut on top of each flattened piece of candy. Refrigerate for at least 2 hours for candy to set. Yield: 20 pieces.

Nutritional Values (per piece)

Calories:	68	Fiber:	.897 g
Carbohydrates:	3.95 g	Protein:	2.39 g
Cholesterol:	0 mg	Sodium:	3.64 mg
Fat:	5.38 g		

Granola Candy

2 cups dry granola
4 tablespoons sugar-free maple syrup
1 cup shredded coconut

In a large bowl, mix the granola and maple syrup. Mix thoroughly.
Granola will be sticky. Add shredded coconut and mix until granola
is thoroughly coated with the coconut and easy to handle. Form into
2" diameter balls. Wrap each piece in waxed paper or colored plastic
wrap. Refrigerate. Yield: 48 pieces.

Nutritional Values (per piece)

Calories:	29.9		Fiber:	.612 g
Carbohydrates:	3.5 g		Protein:	.653 g
Cholesterol:	0 mg		Sodium:	5.01 mg
Fat:	1.66 g			

Fig Sticks

4 cups fresh, whole figs
2 cups almonds
1 cup sesame seeds

Place the figs and almonds in a grinder. Grind together. Mix thoroughly. Place the mixture on waxed paper and roll to ⅛" thick. Cut into rectangular bars 1" wide x 3" long. Place sesame seeds in the center of each bar. Fold sides into the middle, over the sesame seeds. Roll to 1" diameter. Cut ¾" in length. Yield: 80 pieces.

Nutritional Values (per piece)

Calories:	59.1		Fiber:	1.54 g
Carbohydrates:	8.24 g		Protein:	1.49 g
Cholesterol:	0 mg		Sodium:	2.36 mg
Fat:	2.86 g			

Coconut Sticks

4 cups fresh figs
2 cups unsalted almonds
1 cup shredded coconut

Place the fresh figs and almonds in a grinder. Grind together. Mix thoroughly. Place the mixture on waxed paper and roll ⅛" thick. Cut into rectangular bars 1" wide x 3" long. Place the shredded coconut in the center of each bar. Fold sides into the middle, over the shredded coconut. Roll until smooth and cut ½" long. Yield: 80 pieces.

Nutritional Values (per piece)

Calories:	51.6		Fiber:	1.46 g
Carbohydrates:	8.21 g		Protein:	1.03 g
Cholesterol:	0 mg		Sodium:	1.81 mg
Fat:	2.17 g			

⊚

Fruit Bars

1½ pounds fresh, whole figs
1 pound pitted dates
½ pound raisins
¼ pound sunflower seed kernels
½ pound chopped English walnuts
½ pound shredded coconut
2 tablespoons carob powder

Mix together the figs, dates, raisins, sunflower seed kernels and ¼ pound chopped walnuts. Put the entire mixture through a grinder or blender. Mixture will form a paste. Set mixture aside. Place the coconut on a board. Place the ground mixture on top of the coconut. Knead the coconut into the ground mixture. Knead in the carob powder. Shape into 1" diameter x 1½" long bars. Roll in remaining ¼ pound of chopped walnuts. Refrigerate. Yield: 100 pieces.

• *Make carob powder by placing carob in a blender. Blend at high speed until mixture is in a powder form.*

Nutritional Values (per piece)			
Calories:	66.5	Fiber:	1.45 g
Carbohydrates:	10.6 g	Protein:	.968 g
Cholesterol:	0 mg	Sodium:	1.95 mg
Fat:	2.92 g		

Apple-Raisin Surprise

¼ cup raisins
½ cup apple juice
¼ cup pitted dates
1 cup finely chopped almonds
1 cup finely chopped cashews
1 cup shredded coconut

Place the raisins in a small bowl. Add the apple juice. Be sure fruit is covered with the juice. Refrigerate overnight. Then blend the raisins, juice and dates in a blender. Be sure to mix well. Place the mixture in a bowl. Add the almonds and cashews. Mix thoroughly. Shape into 1" diameter balls and roll in shredded coconut. Refrigerate. Yield: 60 pieces.

Nutritional Values (per piece)

Calories:	38.3	Fiber:	.487 g
Carbohydrates:	3.38 g	Protein:	.874 g
Cholesterol:	0 mg	Sodium:	1.55 mg
Fat:	2.65 g		

⊚

Fancy Pecans

1 pound dried figs
¼ pound pecans
¼ pound raisins
¼ pound pitted dried dates

Place the figs, pecans, raisins and dates in a grinder or blender. Once ground, place in a bowl and mix thoroughly. Then place in an 8" x 8" pan. Spread in the pan with spatula or hands. Score top into 1" squares, ½" deep. Refrigerate for at least 2 hours. Cut the squares along scored lines. Yield: 75 pieces.

Nutritional Values (per piece)

Calories:	34.2	Fiber:	.799 g
Carbohydrates:	6.53 g	Protein:	.381 g
Cholesterol:	0 mg	Sodium:	.908 mg
Fat:	1.11 g		

9

Striped Candy Canes

1 large egg white
½ tablespoon cold water
½ teaspoon peppermint extract
2 cups powdered Isomalt®
½ tablespoon red food coloring

Combine egg white, water and peppermint extract in a bowl. Beat
with an electric beater until mixture holds a peak (3 to 4 minutes).
Slowly add the powdered Isomalt®. Continue beating until mixture
is stiff. Place the mixture on a board that has been covered with
powdered Isomalt. Knead until smooth.

Roll half of the mixture into a long roll that is ½ the desired
thickness of the candy canes. Add red food coloring to remaining
mixture. Divide red mixture into 2 halves and roll very thin. Place
red rolls on each side of the white roll. Hold the top of the 3 rolls.
Roll so the red and white alternate like a barber pole. Cut into 7"
lengths. Turn the tops down for the hook of the canes. Set aside on
a rack and allow to dry thoroughly. May be frozen. Yield: 90 canes.

These candy canes are similar to those you purchase in the store!

Nutritional Values (per cane)

Calories:	5.08	Fiber:	0 g
Carbohydrates:	.105 g	Protein:	1.06 g
Cholesterol:	0 mg	Sodium:	16.6 mg
Fat:	0 g		

＠

Old-Fashioned Candy Canes

3 cups Isomalt®
1 cup water
¾ teaspoon peppermint extract
¾ teaspoon red food coloring

Preparation: Prepare molds for hot candy by using aluminum foil. Make a trough that is ½" wide and approximately 18" long. Make another trough that is ¼" wide and approximately 18" long. The ½" trough is for the clear candy liquid. The ¼" wide trough is for the red candy liquid. Oil the troughs well with margarine or vegetable oil.

In a 4-quart heavy saucepan, combine the Isomalt® and water. Stir well. Cook to crack stage. Remove from heat and add peppermint extract. Pour ¾ of mixture into molds of aluminum foil. Add red food coloring to balance of mixture. Pour into aluminum foil mold. As soon as candy is set, place the red stripe on top of the white stripe. Cut to 7" lengths. Fold down sides of mold. Twist the strip. Turn down the tops for the hooks. Do not move until candy has completely set. Yield: 90 canes.

Nutritional Values (per cane)

Calories:	.053	Fiber:	0 g
Carbohydrates:	.014 g	Protein:	0 g
Cholesterol:	0 mg	Sodium:	.076 mg
Fat:	0 g		

⊚

Christmas Trees

¼ cup margarine
2 cups powdered Isomalt®
¼ cup light cream
3 cups shredded coconut
green food coloring
2½ cups carob
⅛ teaspoon artificial sweetener

In a 2-quart saucepan, slowly heat margarine until golden brown. Gradually stir in powdered Isomalt®, cream and coconut. Add green food coloring. Drop by tablespoonfuls onto waxed paper. Chill until easy to handle. Shape into peaks. Melt carob in double boiler. Stir in artificial sweetener. Dip the bottom half of each peak in melted carob. Place on waxed paper to cool. Measures 1" high x ¾" diameter. Yield: 80 pieces.

- *You may place your coconut mixture in a Christmas tree mold. Press mixture into each Christmas tree mold and allow to cool completely. Then dip in melted carob.*

Nutritional Values (per piece)

Calories:	58.1		Fiber:	.282 g
Carbohydrates:	5.15 g		Protein:	1.30 g
Cholesterol:	1.51 mg		Sodium:	.872 mg
Fat:	3.68 g			

After Dinner Mints

4 cups powdered Isomalt®
8 to 10 tablespoons whole milk
green food coloring

Place powdered Isomalt® in a bowl. Use electric mixer. Add milk in small amounts until mixture is stiff. Add mint flavor. Add green food coloring. Roll into 1" diameter balls and flatten with a fork dipped in powdered Isomalt® or place in molds of your choice. Allow to set for at least 2 hours. Yield: 60 pieces.

Nutritional Values (per piece)

Calories:	1.56		Fiber:	0 g
Carbohydrates:	.119 g		Protein:	.084 g
Cholesterol:	.346 mg		Sodium:	1.25 mg
Fat:	.085 g			

Apricot Balls

24 *dried apricots*
1½ cups shredded coconut
2 teaspoons orange juice
⅛ teaspoon artificial sweetener

Wash and dry dried apricots. Put through food chopper together with shredded coconut. Add orange juice and artificial sweetener. Blend well. Shape into 1" diameter balls. If desired, roll in shredded coconut. Yield: 60 pieces.

Nutritional Values (per piece)

Calories:	10.8		Fiber:	.324 g
Carbohydrates:	1.16 g		Protein:	.175 g
Cholesterol:	0 mg		Sodium:	.477 mg
Fat:	.7 g			

Coconut Crisps

2 cups Isomalt®
½ cup whole milk
1½ cups shredded coconut
½ teaspoon vanilla

Heat Isomalt® and milk over low heat, stirring constantly until Isomalt® is dissolved. Increase heat and cook, stirring constantly, until candy reaches a soft ball stage. Remove from heat. Stir in coconut and vanilla. Drop from a teaspoon onto a cookie sheet equal to a 1" diameter ball. Yield: 60 pieces.

Nutritional Values (per piece)

Calories:	8.4	Fiber:	.188 g
Carbohydrates:	.401 g	Protein:	.134 g
Cholesterol:	.277 mg	Sodium:	1.4 mg
Fat:	.738 g		

Coconut Rolls

¹/₄ cup margarine
4 cups powdered Isomalt®
¹/₄ cup light cream
¹/₂ teaspoon vanilla
1 cup shredded coconut

Melt margarine in a 2-quart saucepan. Add powdered Isomalt® alternately with cream and vanilla, stirring well after each addition. Beat until smooth. Sprinkle breadboard or pastry canvas with small amount of powdered Isomalt®. Turn mixture out on board and knead until smooth and glossy, about 10 minutes. Form into 1" diameter balls and roll in coconut. Yield: 60 pieces.

Nutritional Values (per piece)

Calories:	10.9	Fiber:	.031 g
Carbohydrates:	.086 mg	Protein:	.038 g
Cholesterol:	1.1 mg	Sodium:	.43 mg
Fat:	1.18 g		

⊚

Butter Crunch

1 cup margarine
1 cup Isomalt®
2 tablespoons water
1 tablespoon sugar-free maple syrup
¾ cup chopped peanuts
1 cup carob
⅛ teaspoon artificial sweetener

Melt the margarine in a 2-quart saucepan over low heat. Remove from heat. Add Isomalt®. With a wooden spoon, stir the mixture until well blended. Return to low heat. Stir rapidly until thoroughly mixed and beginning to bubble. Add water and sugar-free maple syrup. Mix well. Put in candy thermometer. Keep heat low. Stir frequently until brittle stage (approximately 15 to 20 minutes). Remove from heat at once and take out the candy thermometer.

Sprinkle peanuts over surface and quickly mix in. Pour onto a cookie sheet. With a spatula, spread ¼" thick. Cool to room temperature. As crunch cools, loosen from sheet with spatula 2 or 3 times. Melt the carob and artificial sweetener in a double boiler. Remove from water. Stir well. Spread half of melted carob evenly over crunch. Set aside until firm. Turn onto waxed paper or another cookie sheet carob side down. Spread remaining melted carob evenly. Both sides will be coated. When firm, break candy into pieces of 1" square. Store in lightly covered container in a cool place. Yield: 80 pieces.

Nutritional Values (per piece)

Calories:	28.4		Fiber:	.095 g
Carbohydrates:	.348 g		Protein:	.339 g
Cholesterol:	0 mg		Sodium:	.322 mg
Fat:	2.96 g			

Cherry Fudge

1⅓ tablespoons margarine
2 teaspoons grated orange rind, as desired
1 cup thin cream
3 cups Isomalt®
⅜ teaspoon cream of tartar
3 tablespoons orange juice
1 teaspoon lemon juice
⅔ cup chopped English walnuts
1 3-ounce can or jar of red maraschino cherries

Melt margarine in a 2-quart heavy saucepan. Remove from heat. Add orange rind. Blend thoroughly. Add cream, Isomalt®, cream of tartar and orange juice. Blend thoroughly. Place over low heat. Stir until Isomalt® is dissolved and mixture is boiling gently. Cover. Cook 3 minutes. Remove cover. If crystals form on sides of pan during the cooking process, remove with damp cloth wrapped around tines of a fork. Stir occasionally to soft ball stage. Because this is a very soft fudge, it must be cooked at this low temperature.

Remove from heat. Cool at room temperature until lukewarm. Add lemon juice and nuts. Beat until thick and creamy. This candy requires lots of beating. Spread evenly in a 9" x 9" pan. Cool. Cut in 1" square x ½" deep pieces. Cut red petals from glossy outside peel of cherries. Use three petals to form a flower on each piece of candy. Yield: 90 pieces.

Nutritional Values (per piece)

Calories:	34.6	Fiber:	.043 g
Carbohydrates:	.651 g	Protein:	.231 g
Cholesterol:	.992 mg	Sodium:	1.28 mg
Fat:	3.56 g		

Cherries à la Fudge

4 envelopes unflavored gelatin
½ cup Isomalt®
1½ cups boiling water
2 cups carob
2 cups chopped maraschino cherries

Use a heavy 4-quart saucepan. Mix gelatin with Isomalt®. Add boiling water and stir until gelatin is completely dissolved. Add carob, and stir with a wire whip over low heat until carob is melted and thoroughly blended. Remove from heat. Add maraschino cherries. Mix well. Pour into a 8" x 8" square pan. Cool. Cut into 1" squares, ½" deep. Yield: 80 pieces.

Nutritional Values (per piece)

Calories:	33.5		Fiber:	0 g
Carbohydrates:	4.53 g		Protein:	1.13 g
Cholesterol:	.454 mg		Sodium:	10.9 mg
Fat:	1.25 g			

Creamy Fudge

1 3-ounce package light Philadelphia cream cheese
⅛ teaspoon artificial sweetener
½ teaspoon almond extract
1½ cups chopped almonds
dash of salt or salt substitute

With electric mixer, beat cream cheese until soft and smooth. Slowly blend in artificial sweetener, extract, nuts, and salt or salt substitute. Pour into an 8" x 8" pan. Chill until firm. Cut into 1" squares, ½" deep. Yield: 64 pieces.

Nutritional Values (per piece)

Calories:	19.1	Fiber:	.291 g
Carbohydrates:	.668 g	Protein:	.797 g
Cholesterol:	.234 mg	Sodium:	8.3 mg
Fat:	1.59 g		

Walnut Fudge

3 cups carob
¼ teaspoon artificial sweetener
1 14-ounce can sweet condensed milk (not evapo-
    rated milk)
1 cup chopped walnuts
1½ teaspoon vanilla extract
48 walnut halves

In a heavy 2-quart saucepan, combine the carob, artificial sweetener
and condensed milk. Cook over low heat until carob is completely
melted. Remove from heat. Add chopped walnuts and vanilla extract.
Stir until completely mixed. Pour into a 9" x 9" square pan. Chill in
refrigerator until almost firm. Score the top of the fudge into squares
2" x ½" deep. Place a walnut half on the top of each square. Chill
until firm. Finish cutting into squares. Yield: 48 2"-square pieces.

- *Can be made into smaller pieces. If cut to 1" squares, lower
  nutritional values by 50 percent.*

Nutritional Values (per piece)			
Calories:	137	Fiber:	.302 g
Carbohydrates:	13.5 g	Protein:	3.72 g
Cholesterol:	3.94 mg	Sodium:	11.2 mg
Fat:	7.97 g		

Almond Delight

2 cups blanched almonds
2 cups powdered Isomalt®
Rind of ½ lemon
2 egg whites

Grind almonds very fine through a food grinder or blender. Nuts should be the consistency of dry, white sugar. When you grind the nuts, be sure the nuts are dry. If nuts seem moist and oily, spread them over a shallow pan and dry them in a slow oven, 300° F, before grinding. Put the ground almonds in a large mixing bowl, and stir in Isomalt® and lemon rind. Pound hard with the handle of a wooden spoon. Pound about 5 to 7 minutes to get all the flavor mixed through. Add unbeaten egg whites and knead. Place in an 8" x 8" square pan and refrigerate. Cut into 1" squares, ½" deep. Yield: 60 pieces.

Nutritional Values (per piece)			
Calories:	28.9	Fiber:	.474 g
Carbohydrates:	.909 g	Protein:	1.09 g
Cholesterol:	0 mg	Sodium:	2.15 mg
Fat:	2.54 g		

⊚

Nut Crunch

1¼ cups Isomalt®
¾ cup margarine
¼ cup water
½ cup unblanched almonds
½ teaspoon baking soda
½ cup blanched almonds
⅓ cup carob
⅛ teaspoon artificial sweetener
½ cup finely chopped blanched almonds

In a heavy saucepan mix Isomalt®, margarine, water and unblanched almonds. Boil mixture to brittle stage. Stir occasionally. Stir in baking soda and the blanched almonds. Pour into an 8" x 8" square pan, ¾" deep. Melt carob in double boiler. Stir in artificial sweetener and mix well. Spread sweetened carob evenly on top of candy. Sprinkle with finely chopped nuts. Cool. Break into 1" square pieces. Yield: 80 pieces.

Nutritional Values (per piece)			
Calories:	35.3	Fiber:	.204 g
Carbohydrates:	1.12 g	Protein:	.594 g
Cholesterol:	.085 mg	Sodium:	.315 mg
Fat:	3.32 g		

Pralines

2 cups Isomalt®
1 teaspoon baking soda
1 cup buttermilk
pinch of salt or salt substitute
2 tablespoons margarine
2⅓ cups pecan halves
64 perfect pecan halves (unbroken)

In a large kettle (about 8 quarts), combine Isomalt®, baking soda, buttermilk and salt or salt substitute. Cook over high heat 5 minutes, being sure to stir frequently and to scrape bottom and crevices of kettle. Cook to 234° F on a candy thermometer. Remove from heat. Add margarine and 2⅓ cups pecan halves. Cook, stirring continuously to soft ball stage. Remove and let stand just a minute or 2. Then with a spoon, beat until thickened and creamy. Immediately drop by 2" tablespoonfuls onto waxed paper or a cookie sheet. Dot with perfect pecans. Press pecan into each piece of candy. Yield: 64 pieces.

Nutritional Values (per piece)

Calories:	39.2		Fiber:	.24 g
Carbohydrates:	1.13 g		Protein:	.531 g
Cholesterol:	.134 mg		Sodium:	23.7 mg
Fat:	3.89 g			

Date Roll

8 cups Isomalt®
1 cup heavy cream
1 cup dates
1 cup chopped English walnuts

Cook Isomalt® and cream in a heavy 2-quart saucepan until mixture comes to a boil. Add the dates. Cook until mixture reaches the soft ball stage. Remove from heat. Beat the mixture in the saucepan until creamy. Add the English walnuts and pour onto a damp cloth and mold into a roll 1" in diameter. Keep in cloth in the refrigerator overnight. Remove the candy from the cloth and slice ¾" thick. Yield: 60 pieces.

Nutritional Values (per piece)

Calories:	34.7		Fiber:	.314 g
Carbohydrates:	2.66 g		Protein:	.427 g
Cholesterol:	5.43 mg		Sodium:	1.78 mg
Fat:	2.72 g			

English Toffee

2 cups Isomalt®
1½ cups margarine
2 tablespoons water
2 cups blanched almonds
½ cup grated carob

Combine the Isomalt®, margarine and water in a heavy 2-quart saucepan. Cook over low heat so mixture will not burn. Cook until margarine is melted. Stir mixture occasionally. Add the almonds. Continue cooking slowly without stirring to 280° or to a hard crack stage. Pour into a shallow pan or onto a cookie sheet to ½" thickness. Sprinkle with the grated carob. Break into 1" square pieces. Yield: 80 pieces.

Nutritional Values (per piece)			
Calories:	57.9	Fiber:	.338 g
Carbohydrates:	1.52 g	Protein:	.942 g
Cholesterol:	.113 mg	Sodium:	.484 mg
Fat:	5.58 g		

Sweet Nuts

1 cup Isomalt®
¼ cup water
1 teaspoon vanilla
1 cup chopped English walnuts

Boil Isomalt® and water until mixture threads from a spoon or reaches a hard crack stage. Remove from heat. Add vanilla and English walnuts. Stir well. Pour onto a cookie sheet to ½" deep. Spread out and allow to cool completely. Break or cut into 1" square pieces. Yield: 100 pieces.

• *Other nuts may be used, such as almonds, cashews or peanuts.*

Nutritional Values (per piece)

Calories:	6.51		Fiber:	.045 g
Carbohydrates:	.184 g		Protein:	.143 g
Cholesterol:	0 mg		Sodium:	.101 mg
Fat:	.619 g			

ↄ

_____

Potato Bon Bons

6 potatoes
1 teaspoon vanilla
1 cup powdered Isomalt®
2 cups carob

Peel potatoes and boil. Pour off water and mash potatoes thoroughly.
Add vanilla. Mix thoroughly. Add powdered Isomalt®. Mix well.
Mixture will hold its shape. Shape mixture into 1" diameter balls
and place on a cookie sheet. Place carob in double boiler and melt.
Dip each potato ball in melted carob. Place on waxed paper to cool.
Yield: 75 pieces.

Nutritional Values (per piece)

Calories:	27.3		Fiber:	.141 g
Carbohydrates:	4.24 g		Protein:	.748 g
Cholesterol:	.302 mg		Sodium:	.541 mg
Fat:	.842 g			

Cinnamon Bon Bons

1½ cups Isomalt®
½ cup evaporated milk
1 tablespoon margarine
½ teaspoon cream of tartar
¼ teaspoon salt or salt substitute
1 teaspoon vanilla
1 cup cinnamon
1 cup chopped English walnuts

Cook Isomalt®, milk, margarine, cream of tartar and salt or salt substitute to boiling point, stirring constantly. Continue cooking, stirring
occasionally until the mixture forms a soft ball. Remove from heat.
Cool to lukewarm. Add vanilla. Beat until creamy and stiff. Shape
with fingers into 1" diameter balls. Then shape each ball to resemble
potatoes. Roll in cinnamon. Insert 3 pieces of walnuts in each piece
of candy to look like the "eyes" of a potato. Yield: 80 pieces.

Nutritional Values (per piece)

Calories:	37.9	Fiber:	.2 g
Carbohydrates:	4.44 g	Protein:	1.04 g
Cholesterol:	.341 mg	Sodium:	2.5 mg
Fat:	1.86 g		

Cream Delight

2 cups carob
⅛ teaspoon artificial sweetener
¼ cup heavy whipping cream

Melt the carob and artificial sweetener in a double boiler. Remove the top portion of the double boiler that contains the carob and set aside. Heat the whipping cream in a separate saucepan until boiling. Gradually pour the boiling cream into the melted carob, beating constantly. Candy will become dark and appear glossy. Place the candy back on top of double boiler. Cook over medium heat. Stir constantly until candy is very thick. Remove from heat. Cool candy until it can be handled. Place on waxed paper and spread to ½" thick. Cut in 1" squares or use candy cutters or molds. Yield: 60 pieces.

Nutritional Values (per piece)

Calories:	25.8	Fiber:	0 g
Carbohydrates:	2.62 g	Protein:	.723 g
Cholesterol:	1.74 mg	Sodium:	.373 mg
Fat:	1.41 g		

Cocoa Balls

¾ cup cocoa
1¾ cups powdered Isomalt®
1 cup chopped walnuts or pecans
½ cup sweet condensed milk
1 tablespoon vanilla

Mix ½ cup cocoa and 1½ cup powdered Isomalt®. Add chopped walnuts or pecans and mix thoroughly. Add condensed milk and vanilla. Shape into 1" diameter balls. Combine the remaining powdered Isomalt® and cocoa in a separate bowl. Roll the balls in the mixture until completely coated. Chill. Yield: 75 pieces.

Nutritional Values (per piece)

Calories:	19.5		Fiber:	.36 g
Carbohydrates:	1.87 g		Protein:	.453 g
Cholesterol:	.693 mg		Sodium:	2.79 mg
Fat:	1.37 g			

Buckeyes

½ cup margarine
1 pound peanut butter
4 cups powdered Isomalt®
1 cup carob chips

Cream together the margarine and peanut butter. Add powdered Iso-malt® gradually and blend. The mixture will be crumbly. Shape into 1" diameter balls. Place a toothpick in each ball. Melt the carob in a double boiler. Dip each ball in the melted carob. Place on waxed paper. Chill until firm. Yield: 75 pieces.

Nutritional Values (per piece)

Calories:	61.2		Fiber:	.399 g
Carbohydrates:	2.63 g		Protein:	2.1 g
Cholesterol:	.242 mg		Sodium:	1.06 mg
Fat:	5.06 g			

Almond Balls

1 package dry yeast
1/4 cup warm water
1 cup scalded whole milk (no canned milk, please!)
1 teaspoon artificial sweetener
1/3 cup margarine
1/2 teaspoon salt substitute
4 cups sifted all-purpose flour
3 large eggs, well beaten
1/4 cup melted margarine
1 cup chopped almonds

Preheat oven to 300° F. Place the yeast in the warm water. Set aside. In a 1-quart heavy saucepan, scald the milk. Blend in the artificial sweetener, 1/3 cup margarine and the salt substitute. Stir well and continue cooking until the artificial sweetener is dissolved. Remove from heat. Add the eggs and yeast mixture. Pour into a large bowl and add the flour. Beat well. Place the mixture on a floured board and knead until smooth. Shape into a large ball. Place in a bowl and cover with a cloth. Let stand until mixture rises to double its size. Punch it down and let it rise again to twice its size. Then shape the dough into 1" diameter balls. Melt a 1/4 cup of margarine. Place the melted margarine in a bowl. Place the chopped almonds in another bowl. Dip the balls into the melted margarine and then into the almonds. Coat well. Place on a cookie sheet. Cook in the oven for 15 to 20 minutes. Remove and place on waxed paper to cool. Yield: 75 pieces.

Nutritional Values (per piece)

Calories:	72.2	Fiber:	.631 g
Carbohydrates:	9.62 g	Protein:	2.08 g
Cholesterol:	7.63 mg	Sodium:	4.61 mg
Fat:	2.9 g		

Sweet Fruit

½ cup dried prunes
½ cup dried apricots
½ cup raisins
½ cup chopped cashew nuts
½ cup artificial sweetener

Rinse the prunes, apricots and raisins thoroughly. Let dry completely. Chop the prunes, apricots and raisins into very fine pieces. A food processor is faster; otherwise, use a sharp knife on a wooden cutting board. Mix the chopped nuts and fruit together. Shape into 1" diameter balls. Place artificial sweetener in another bowl. Roll the small balls in powdered artificial sweetener. Place on waxed paper to dry. Yield: 50 pieces.

Nutritional Values (per piece)

Calories:	18.4	Fiber:	.329 g
Carbohydrates:	3.19 g	Protein:	.338 g
Cholesterol:	0 mg	Sodium:	.499 mg
Fat:	.661 g		

Date Balls

3 tablespoons margarine
2 eggs, well beaten
⅔ cups Isomalt®
1 cup chopped dates
2 cups dry rice cereal
1 cup chopped English walnuts
1 teaspoon vanilla extract
1 cup shredded coconut

In a heavy 2-quart saucepan melt the margarine. Set aside. In a bowl, beat the eggs and Isomalt® together. Add the chopped dates. Pour this mixture into the saucepan with the melted margarine. Cook over low heat, stirring constantly, until the mixture is very thick. Remove from heat. Add rice cereal, nuts and vanilla extract. Allow mixture to cool to lukewarm, or until it can be handled comfortably. Form into 1" balls. Roll the balls in the shredded coconut. Refrigerate to set. Yield: 80 pieces.

Nutritional Values (per piece)

Calories:	27.5	Fiber:	.338 g
Carbohydrates:	2.7 g	Protein:	.41 g
Cholesterol:	5.33 mg	Sodium:	5.76 mg
Fat:	1.83 g		

Candied Prunes

80 dried, pitted prunes
1 cup water
¼ cup cider vinegar
2 sticks cinnamon
¼ teaspoon mint extract

In a heavy 4-quart saucepan cook the prunes, water, vinegar and cinnamon sticks. Bring the mixture to a boil. Continue boiling until the prunes are tender. Remove from heat. Add the mint extract. Stir well. Let stand for 12 hours in the refrigerator. Drain prunes. Keep in a cool, dry place. Yield: 80 pieces.

Nutritional Values (per piece)

Calories:	13.7		Fiber:	.524 g
Carbohydrates:	3.6 g		Protein:	.148 g
Cholesterol:	0 mg		Sodium:	.234 mg
Fat:	.029 g			

🌀

Vanilla Raisin Clusters

1 cup carob
⅛ teaspoon artificial sweetener
1 teaspoon vanilla extract
2 cups raisins

In a double boiler melt the carob. Remove from heat. Add the artificial sweetener and vanilla extract. Stir well. Add raisins. Drop by 2" square shaped spoonfuls onto waxed paper or into candy cups. Allow to cool thoroughly. Yield: 60 pieces.

Nutritional Values (per piece)			
Calories:	32.5	Fiber:	.168 g
Carbohydrates:	5.92 g	Protein:	.718 g
Cholesterol:	.302 mg	Sodium:	.581 mg
Fat:	.854 g		

Filled Fruit

12 dried apricots
1 3-ounce package light Philadelphia cream cheese
¼ cup unsalted margarine
1 teaspoon vanilla extract
⅛ teaspoon artificial sweetener

Place apricots in scalding water. Let soak until soft. Remove and let dry on a wire rack. While fruit is drying, make cream cheese filling by mixing together the cream cheese, margarine and vanilla extract. Add the artificial sweetener. Mix well. Place 1 teaspoon of mixture in the center of each apricot. Yield: 12 pieces.

Nutritional Values (per piece)

Calories:	53.1		Fiber:	.465 g
Carbohydrates:	3.15 g		Protein:	1.39 g
Cholesterol:	1.25 mg		Sodium:	42.8 mg
Fat:	3.9 g			

Orange Sticks

⅓ cup orange juice
⅓ cup dry rolled oats
⅓ cup margarine
2 cups powdered Isomalt®
3 tablespoons cocoa
⅔ cup chopped walnuts
⅔ cup raisins
⅔ cup shredded coconut
¼ teaspoon ground nutmeg
¼ teaspoon ground cinnamon

In a large bowl, mix the orange juice and rolled oats. Let mixture set for 1 hour. Then place the margarine in a small saucepan. Melt over low heat. Set aside. Add the powdered Isomalt®, cocoa, walnuts, raisins, shredded coconut, nutmeg, cinnamon and margarine to the bowl containing the orange juice and rolled oats mixture. Stir well. Place in the refrigerator for at least 1 hour. Remove and form into sticks ¼" wide x ½" long x ¾" thick. Place on waxed paper or wire rack to dry. Yield: 75 pieces.

Nutritional Values (per piece)

Calories:	24.3		Fiber:	.219 g
Carbohydrates:	2.04 g		Protein:	.44 g
Cholesterol:	.048 mg		Sodium:	4.37 mg
Fat:	1.76 g			

Pumpkin Squares

1 cup cooked and mashed pumpkin
¼ teaspoon pumpkin pie spice
1 3-ounce package cream cheese
2 cups powdered Isomalt®

Cook pumpkin until partially firm. If you overcook the pumpkin, your candy will not be firm. Mash pumpkin well. The pumpkin will still hold its shape. Place pumpkin, pumpkin pie spice and cream cheese in a bowl. Blend well. Add powdered Isomalt® ½ cup at a time and stir well. Mixture will be thick. Place in an 8" x 8" square pan. Refrigerate overnight. Cut into 1" squares, ½" deep. Yield: 80 pieces.

Nutritional Values (per piece)

Calories:	1.57	Fiber:	.028 g
Carbohydrates:	.191 g	Protein:	.172 g
Cholesterol:	.187 mg	Sodium:	6.4 mg
Fat:	.003 g		

Bon Bons

2 cups carob
1 teaspoon artificial sweetener
1 pint ice milk
80 small candy paper cups

Melt carob in a double boiler. Remove from heat. Add artificial sweetener and mix well. Cool to the point mixture can be spooned into paper cups. Fill each cup half full. Add small scoop of ice milk. Spoon more carob mixture over the top of the ice milk. Be sure mixture covers the ice milk. Immediately place in the freezer. Yield: 80 pieces.

- *Be sure ice milk is frozen solid. If not, the ice milk will melt before you can finish spooning the melted carob over the top and placing in the freezer.*

Nutritional Values (per piece)

Calories:	31.4		Fiber:	.003 g
Carbohydrates:	3.86 g		Protein:	.968 g
Cholesterol:	.916 mg		Sodium:	2.81 mg
Fat:	1.39 g			

๑

Frosted Fruit

45 strawberries
1 egg white
2 tablespoons water
1 cup powdered Isomalt®

Wash strawberries and let dry. Place egg white and water in bowl. Beat lightly. Place the powdered Isomalt® in another bowl. Dip strawberries in egg white mixture. Then dip in powdered Isomalt®. Repeat to thicken the coating. Place on a baking sheet lined with waxed paper. Allow to dry thoroughly. Store in airtight container in the refrigerator. Yield: 45 pieces.

- *Other fruits may be used. If a fruit such as dates or prunes are used, the fruit can be dipped and placed on a cookie sheet lined with cooking paper. Then place in an oven heated to 170° until dry. Remove from oven and cool. Store in airtight container in the refrigerator.*

Nutritional Values (per piece)			
Calories:	3.7	Fiber:	.154 g
Carbohydrates:	.721 g	Protein:	.203 g
Cholesterol:	0 mg	Sodium:	2.32 mg
Fat:	.037 g		

Dipped Pecans

5 cups powdered Isomalt®
½ cup margarine
1 egg white, stiffly beaten
1½ teaspoons vanilla extract
2 cups carob
1 teaspoon artificial sweetener
80 pecan halves

Combine 2½ cups powdered Isomalt® with margarine in a bowl. Combine the remaining 2½ cups powdered Isomalt® with stiffly beaten egg white in another bowl. Add the contents from the first bowl to the egg white mixture in the second bowl. Cream mixture together. Add vanilla extract. Knead until candy is light and creamy. Roll into a ball. Cover with waxed paper. Store in airtight container in the refrigerator for 24 hours to ripen. Remove and roll into 1" diameter balls. Melt carob and artificial sweetener in double boiler. Dip balls in melted carob. Place on cookie sheet to cool. While cooling, flatten with pecan half on each ball. Yield: 80 pieces.

Nutritional Values (per piece)

Calories:	55.3		Fiber:	.125 g
Carbohydrates:	3.62 g		Protein:	1.13 g
Cholesterol:	.454 mg		Sodium:	1.22 mg
Fat:	4.21 g			

Pretzels

4 cups carob chips
2 cups sifted cocoa

In a double boiler, melt the carob. Place in a pastry decorating bag. Squeeze out in a pretzel design onto a sheet of waxed paper in 1" diameter, ⅛" thick. Let set. Once set, dip in sifted cocoa. Place again on waxed paper to dry. Keep in a well sealed container away from heat and moisture. Yield: 60 pieces.

Nutritional Values (per piece)

Calories:	71.6	Fiber:	0 g
Carbohydrates:	8.3 g	Protein:	2.25 g
Cholesterol:	1.21 mg	Sodium:	0 mg
Fat:	3.33 g		

OTHER SWEET TREATS

Treat-Making Tips

This section contains wonderful diabetic treats that are not candy, but do feed the soul and take care of that marvelous "sweet tooth" in a healthy and satisfying way. If you desire to make large batches of any recipe in this section, simply increase the amounts used in each recipe to suit your needs. This is especially easy and helpful for serving large groups.

When you are using the ingredients in these recipes, you will find that everyday items are used. There is nothing exotic in these recipes. The results can be exotic in their appeal and taste, however.

Below are some hints when using the ingredients:

CAKE FLOUR: You may use cake flour in your recipes rather than bleached or unbleached flour where "flour" is called for. However, cake flour will change the nutritional values. When a recipe calls for "cake flour," please use that particular flour in that recipe and do not substitute an all-purpose white flour.

DIABETIC OR NO-SUGAR INGREDIENTS: When called for, please use the specified diabetic or no-sugar ingredient. Any substitution will change the nutritional values.

FAT CONTENT: The nutritional values note fat content per recipe. This is the *total* fat content and it includes saturated fat, polyunsaturated fat, and monounsaturated fat.

FLOUR: Flour used herein is an all-purpose white flour. You may use either bleached or unbleached flour. This is your choice and will not change the taste of your recipe. Flour measurements are sifted measurements.

NUTRITIONAL VALUES: Nutritional values are given on the specific recipe with the specific ingredients. Any change of ingredients will change the nutritional values.

POLYUNSATURATED OIL: Any oil used in these recipes is polyunsaturated oil to give the best for diabetic needs and healthy eating.

SUGAR SUBSTITUTE: The recipes in this section that call for sugar substitute use granulated or powdered sugar substitutes. Do not use liquid sugar substitutes. Using the same measurement as a granulated or powdered sugar substitute, your recipe will be too sweet.

_9_C_9_C

Cakes

White Frosting

1 8-ounce package Philadelphia light cream cheese
¼ cup plain yogurt
1 teaspoon vanilla extract

Place the cream cheese in a small bowl. Beat until smooth. Add the plain yogurt and vanilla extract. Beat until smooth and thick. Yield: 2 cups of frosting.

To flavor white frosting use any of the following:
  ¼ cup shredded coconut
  ⅓ cup carob powder
  3 tablespoons dry buttermilk
  Any flavor of extract: almond, orange, lemon, rum, peppermint
  Any of your favorite fruits, chopped fine: strawberries, cherries, blueberries, oranges, lemons, apples, tangerines, etc.
  Use your imagination and enjoy a variety of flavors on your favorite cake.

Nutritional Values (2 cups)

Calories:	234	Fiber:	0 g
Carbohydrates:	12.6 g	Protein:	35.5 g
Cholesterol:	41 mg	Sodium:	1406 mg
Fat:	.11 g		

Blueberry Cake

3 large eggs
½ cup unsalted margarine
1 cup pure orange juice
2½ cups cake flour
1 teaspoon baking soda
2 teaspoons baking powder
1 cup shredded coconut
1 cup fresh or frozen blueberries (thawed and
  drained)

Preheat oven to 350° F. In a large bowl mix the eggs, margarine and orange juice. Beat well. Add the cake flour, baking soda and baking powder. Beat well. Stir in the coconut and blueberries. Mix well with a spoon. Place the mixture in a nonstick 9" x 13" cake pan. Bake 25 to 30 minutes. When cool, frost with White Frosting (page 83). Yield: 32 pieces.

Nutritional Values (per serving)

Calories:	68.6	Fiber:	.684 g
Carbohydrates:	7.96 g	Protein:	1.47 g
Cholesterol:	20 mg	Sodium:	19.8 mg
Fat:	3.53 g		

Cherry Cheesecake

1 Graham Cracker Crust (page 118)
1 13-ounce can evaporated skim milk
2 tablespoons cornstarch
¼ cup sugar substitute
1 3-ounce package Philadelphia light cream cheese
¼ cup pure lemon juice
1½ teaspoons vanilla extract
1 1-pound can unsweetened cherries with juice
2 tablespoons cornstarch
2 tablespoons sugar substitute

Prepare the graham cracker crust and place in a 9" pie pan. Set aside. In a small saucepan, cook the evaporated skim milk and cornstarch until thick. Remove from heat and add ¼ cup sugar substitute. Stir well. Set aside to cool. In a small bowl, place the cream cheese and beat well. Add the mixture from the small saucepan. Beat well. Add the lemon juice and vanilla extract. Beat until well blended. Pour into the graham cracker crust. Place in the refrigerator for 2 hours. While cooling, prepare cherry topping. Drain the cherries but save the cherry juice. Place the cherry juice and cornstarch in a small saucepan. Cook over medium heat, stirring constantly. Mixture will become thick and clear. Add the cherries and the 2 tablespoons sugar substitute. Stir well. Set aside to cool. When cool, spread over the cream cheese. Refrigerate for 1 hour. Yield: 10 pieces.

Nutritional Values (per serving)

Calories:	66.3	Fiber:	.416 g
Carbohydrates:	12 g	Protein:	4.37 g
Cholesterol:	2.82 mg	Sodium:	96.8 mg
Fat:	.129 g		

Applesauce-Pineapple Cake

2 cups dietetic canned applesauce
2 cups dietetic canned crushed pineapple
1 cup unsalted margarine, melted
1 sugar-free yellow cake mix
1½ cups chopped English walnuts

Preheat oven to 350° F. In a nonstick 9" x 13" cake pan, place the ingredients as follows: Spread the applesauce on the bottom of the cake pan. Spread evenly. On top of the applesauce, pour the crushed pineapple and spread evenly but do not mix. On top of the pineapple, place the melted margarine. On top of the margarine, place the yellow cake mix and cover evenly. Do not mix. On top of the yellow cake mix, spread the English walnuts. Bake for 60 minutes. Remove to a wire rack to cool. Frost with White Frosting (page 83). Yield: 32 2" square pieces.

Nutritional Values (per serving)

Calories:	105	Fiber:	.544 g
Carbohydrates:	9.58 g	Protein:	1.27 g
Cholesterol:	.177 mg	Sodium:	84 mg
Fat:	7.29 g		

Vanilla Cake

½ cup diet margarine
¾ cup sugar substitute
2 teaspoons vanilla extract
⅓ cup egg whites
2 cups cake flour
2 teaspoons baking powder
2 tablespoons instant dry milk
½ cup lukewarm water
½ cup slivered almonds

Preheat oven to 350° F. In a large bowl, cream together the margarine, sugar substitute, and vanilla extract. Add the egg whites and beat well. In a separate small bowl, mix together with a fork the flour, baking powder and dry milk. Add the dry mixed ingredients to the large bowl. Mix well. Add the lukewarm water and beat well. Place the batter in a 9" x 9" square nonstick cake pan. Sprinkle the slivered almonds on top of the batter. Bake for 30 to 35 minutes. Place on a wire rack to cool. Cut into 2" squares. Yield: 32 pieces.

Nutritional Values (per serving)

Calories:	47.8		Fiber:	.302 g
Carbohydrates:	5.15 g		Protein:	1.21 g
Cholesterol:	0 mg		Sodium:	17.2 mg
Fat:	2.53 g			

Mock Chocolate Cake

1¾ cups flour
⅓ cup carob powder
¾ cup sugar substitute
2 tablespoons instant dry milk
½ teaspoon cinnamon
¼ teaspoon salt substitute
2 teaspoons baking powder
1 cup lukewarm water
2 large eggs
⅓ cup polyunsaturated oil
1½ teaspoons vanilla extract

Preheat oven to 350° F. In a large bowl mix together with a fork the flour, carob powder, sugar substitute, dry milk, cinnamon, salt substitute and baking powder. In a separate small bowl, place the lukewarm water, eggs, polyunsaturated oil and vanilla extract. Use a wire whisk and briskly beat the ingredients until well mixed and frothy. Add the frothy mixture to the large bowl of mixed dry ingredients. Place the batter in a 9" x 9" square nonstick cake pan. Bake 30 to 35 minutes. Cool on a wire rack. Cut in 2" squares. Yield: 32 servings.

Nutritional Values (per serving)

Calories:	54.9	Fiber:	.651 g
Carbohydrates:	6.47 g	Protein:	1.24 g
Cholesterol:	13.4 mg	Sodium:	6.15 mg
Fat:	2.66 g		

❾

Orange Pound Cake

½ cup diet margarine
⅓ cup sugar substitute
3 teaspoons orange extract
4 large eggs
1¾ cups flour
1½ teaspoons baking powder
¼ teaspoon salt substitute

Preheat oven to 350° F. In a large bowl, place the margarine, sugar substitute and orange extract. Beat until well blended. Add eggs to the blended mixture. Beat well. In a small bowl, mix together with a fork the flour, baking powder and salt substitute. Add to the mixture in the large bowl, a little at a time, beating well. Place the batter in a nonstick loaf pan 9" x 5". Bake for 1 hour. Remove to a wire rack and allow to cool completely. Cut cake ½" thick. Yield: 18 pieces.

Nutritional Values (per serving)

Calories:	82.9	Fiber:	.398 g
Carbohydrates:	9.61 g	Protein:	2.67 g
Cholesterol:	47.3 mg	Sodium:	36.8 mg
Fat:	3.68 g		

Chocolate Cake

1 cup flour
½ cup sugar substitute
3 tablespoons carob powder
1½ teaspoons baking powder
½ cup evaporated skim milk
2 tablespoons polyunsaturated oil
1 teaspoon vanilla extract
1 cup brown sugar substitute
½ cup carob powder
1¾ cups boiling water

Preheat oven to 350° F. Use a 9" x 9" square nonstick cake pan. In the pan, place the flour, sugar substitute, 3 tablespoons carob powder, baking powder and evaporated skim milk. Mix well with a wooden spoon so as not to scratch the nonstick surface of your cake pan. When well blended, add the polyunsaturated oil and vanilla extract, and stir until well blended. In a small bowl, mix the 1 cup brown sugar and ½ cup carob powder together. Sprinkle the blended mixture over the batter in the cake pan. Pour the boiling water on top of the mixture. Do NOT stir. Bake for 40 minutes. Yield: 16 2"-square pieces.

Nutritional Values (per serving)

Calories:	54.3	Fiber:	.736 g
Carbohydrates:	7.95 g	Protein:	1.47 g
Cholesterol:	.287 mg	Sodium:	9.74 mg
Fat:	1.8 g		

❍

Lemon Cheesecake

1 Graham Cracker Crust (page 118)
1 8-ounce package Philadelphia light cream cheese
2 cups cold milk
1 3-ounce package sugar-free instant lemon pud-
  ding mix
½ teaspoon grated lemon peel

Prepare graham cracker crust. Place in a 9" x 9" pie pan. Set aside.
In a large bowl, place the cream cheese. Beat well. Gradually add
milk ½ cup at a time. Beat well. Add the lemon pudding mix. Beat
well. Add the lemon peel and beat well. Continue beating until mixture is thick. Pour into the prepared graham cracker crust. Refrigerate
for at least 3 hours or place in freezer until ready to serve. The
cheesecake thaws quickly. Yield: 10 wedges.

Nutritional Values (per serving)

Calories:	121	Fiber:	.364 g
Carbohydrates:	17.9 g	Protein:	4.73 g
Cholesterol:	1.84 mg	Sodium:	189 mg
Fat:	3.54 g		

Peach Upside-Down Cake

¾ cup packed brown sugar substitute
1 tablespoon polyunsaturated oil
2 teaspoons water
1 cup frozen sliced peaches, thawed and drained
1 cup fresh cranberries
¾ cup sugar substitute
¼ cup skim milk
¼ cup plain nonfat yogurt
3 tablespoons polyunsaturated oil
1 teaspoon vanilla extract
1¼ cup sifted cake flour
½ teaspoon baking powder
⅛ teaspoon salt substitute
2 egg whites

Preheat oven to 350° F. In a small saucepan, combine the brown sugar substitute, 1 tablespoon polyunsaturated oil and water. Stir well. Cook over medium heat until the brown sugar substitute dissolves. Stir occasionally. Pour the mixture into a 9" x 9" square nonstick cake pan. Arrange the peach slices in the bottom of the pan. Place the cranberries over the peach slices. Set aside. In a small bowl, combine ¾ cup sugar substitute, skim milk, yogurt, 3 tablespoons polyunsaturated oil and vanilla extract. Stir well with a wire whisk.

In a large bowl, combine the sifted cake flour, baking powder and salt. Stir well with a fork. Add the ingredients from the small bowl to the large bowl, a little at a time. Beat until well blended. Set aside. Place the egg whites in a small bowl and beat until stiff peaks form. Fold the egg white mixture into the large bowl of mixed ingredients. Pour the batter on top of ingredients in the cake pan. Bake for 40 minutes. Immediately invert the cake onto a serving platter. Allow to cool. Yield: 32 ½" square x 2" thick pieces.

Nutritional Values (per serving)

Calories:	23.9		Fiber:	.259 g
Carbohydrates:	4.16 g		Protein:	.752 g
Cholesterol:	.069 mg		Sodium:	5.98 mg
Fat:	.476 g			

☺

Almond Pound Cake

⅔ cup sugar substitute
⅔ cup prune purée (page 135)
¼ cup diet margarine
½ teaspoon almond extract
½ teaspoon vanilla extract
2 egg whites
1 egg
1¾ cups flour
2 teaspoons baking powder
½ teaspoon ground allspice
⅛ teaspoon salt substitute
⅓ cup skim milk

Preheat oven to 350° F. In a large bowl, mix the sugar substitute, prune purée, margarine, almond extract, vanilla extract and the 2 egg whites. Beat well. Add the egg. Beat well. In another bowl, place the flour, baking powder, ground allspice and salt substitute. Stir with a fork to mix. Then begin adding the dry mixture to the mixture in the large bowl. Alternate this with the skim milk. Keep adding the ingredients until all are well blended. Pour the batter into an 8½" x 4½" loaf pan. Bake for 1 hour. Let cool to warm on a wire rack. Serve with the Lemon Sauce (below). Yield: 20 servings 1" thick x 4½".

Lemon Sauce

1 cup apple cider
½ cup sugar substitute
1 tablespoon cornstarch
⅛ teaspoon salt substitute
1 teaspoon grated lemon rind
¼ cup fresh lemon juice

In a small saucepan, cook the apple cider, sugar substitute, cornstarch and salt substitute. Stir with a wire whisk until well blended. Bring mixture to a boil for 1 minute or until thickened. Be sure to stir constantly. Remove from heat. Add the grated lemon rind and lemon juice. Pour over each serving of pound cake. Serve immediately.

Nutritional Values (per serving)

Calories:	56.8		Fiber:	.358 g
Carbohydrates:	8.82 g		Protein:	1.95 g
Cholesterol:	10.7 mg		Sodium:	21.3 mg
Fat:	1.47 g			

Cranberry Banana Loaf Cake

2 cups flour
⅔ cup firmly packed brown sugar substitute
⅓ cup sugar substitute
2 teaspoons baking powder
⅛ teaspoon salt substitute
2 cups mashed very ripe bananas
¼ cup water
¼ cup polyunsaturated oil
1 teaspoon vanilla extract
3 egg whites, lightly beaten
¾ cup chopped cranberries
¼ cup chopped walnuts

Preheat oven to 350° F. In a large bowl, mix well the flour, brown sugar substitute, sugar substitute, baking powder and salt substitute. In a separate bowl, mix together the mashed bananas, water, polyunsaturated oil, vanilla, egg whites and chopped cranberries. Add the mixture, a little at a time, to the large bowl of dry ingredients. Mix very well. Pour the batter into a 9" x 5" nonstick loaf pan. Sprinkle the chopped walnuts over the top. Bake for 65 minutes. Remove from the oven and place on a wire rack to cool. Yield: 32 ½" thick slices.

Nutritional Values (per piece)

Calories:	64.4	Fiber:	.659 g
Carbohydrates:	9.73 g	Protein:	1.28 g
Cholesterol:	0 mg	Sodium:	3.32 mg
Fat:	2.43 g		

⊚

_____

Cranberry Loaf Cake

2 cups flour
²/₃ cup firmly packed brown sugar substitute
¹/₃ cup sugar substitute
2 teaspoons baking powder
¹/₈ teaspoon salt substitute
1³/₄ teaspoons pumpkin pie spice
1 cup unsweetened canned pumpkin
¹/₄ cup water
¹/₄ cup polyunsaturated oil
1¹/₂ teaspoons vanilla extract
3 egg whites, lightly beaten
³/₄ cup chopped cranberries
¹/₄ cup chopped pecans

Preheat oven to 350° F. In a large bowl, mix well the flour, brown sugar substitute, sugar substitute, baking powder, salt substitute and pumpkin pie spice. In a separate bowl, mix together the unsweetened canned pumpkin, water, polyunstaurated oil, vanilla, egg whites and chopped cranberries. Add the mixture, a little at a time, to the large bowl of dry ingredients. Mix very well. Pour the batter into a 9" x 5" nonstick loaf pan. Sprinkle the chopped pecans over the top. Bake for 65 minutes. Remove from the oven and place on a wire rack to cool. Yield: 32 ½" thick slices.

Nutritional Values (per piece)

Calories:	56	Fiber:	.804 g
Carbohydrates:	7.22 g	Protein:	1.06 g
Cholesterol:	0 mg	Sodium:	.957 mg
Fat:	2.46 g		

Carrot Cake

2½ cups flour
1 cup sugar substitute
2 teaspoons baking soda
2 teaspoons ground cinnamon
2 8-ounce cans dietetic crushed pineapple, undrained
¼ cup skim milk
4 egg whites
2 teaspoons vanilla extract
2 cups grated carrots
½ cup golden raisins

Preheat oven to 325° F. In a large bowl, place the flour, sugar substitute, baking soda and cinnamon. Mix well. Add the canned pineapple and the juice, skim milk, egg whites and vanilla extract. Beat well. Fold in the carrots and raisins until well mixed. Use a 9" x 13" nonstick pan. Bake at 325° F for 35 minutes. Check with a wood toothpick. When the toothpick inserted into the middle of the cake comes out clean, the cake is done. Remove and set aside. Let the cake cool to room temperature. While cake is cooling, prepare the icing.

Icing

8 ounces nonfat cream cheese
1 cup nonfat ricotta cheese
½ cup powdered Isomalt®

Place all ingredients in a small bowl. Beat until smooth. Frost the top of the cake. Cake will be 2½" thick. Cut into 3" squares. Yield: 50 pieces.

Nutritional Values (per piece)

Calories:	35.9		Fiber:	.496 g
Carbohydrates:	8.02 g		Protein:	.829 g
Cholesterol:	.022 mg		Sodium:	52.9 mg
Fat:	.095 g			

🌀

Crunchy Chocolate Cupcakes

1½ cups flour
¾ cup wheat germ
¼ cup sugar substitute
1 tablespoon baking powder
1 cup skim milk
¼ cup diet margarine, melted
1 egg
1 cup carob chips

Preheat oven to 400° F. Place paper cups in muffin tins and set aside. In a large bowl, mix the flour, wheat germ, sugar substitute and baking powder together with a fork. Set aside. In a small bowl, mix together the skim milk, diet margarine and egg. Beat well. Slowly add the mixture from the small bowl to the large bowl. Beat well. Add carob chips and mix well. Place batter in cupcake paper cups in muffin tins. Fill the cups half full. Bake 20 to 25 minutes. Yield: 24 1½" diameter 2" deep cupcakes.

Nutritional Values (per serving)

Calories:	96.7		Fiber:	.721 g
Carbohydrates:	13.5 g		Protein:	3.3 g
Cholesterol:	.94 mg		Sodium:	14.6 mg
Fat:	3.4 g			

@

Date Cupcakes

2 cups flour
1 teaspoon baking powder
1 teaspoon baking soda
¼ teaspoon salt substitute
2 teaspoons grated orange rind
½ cup sugar substitute
1 medium sized orange, peeled and sectioned
½ cup diet margarine
½ cup chopped dates
½ cup orange juice
1 egg

Preheat oven to 400° F. Place the flour, baking powder, baking soda, salt substitute, grated orange rind and sugar substitute in a large bowl. Mix well. In a blender, place the orange sections, diet margarine, dates, orange juice and egg. Blend at medium speed until ingredients are well blended but lumpy. Add the blended ingredients to the mixture in the bowl. You may use paper cupcake cups if you so desire. Spoon the batter into the paper cupcake holders or directly into your muffin tin. Fill half full. Bake in the oven for 15 minutes. Yield: 24 cupcakes, 2" diameter x 1½" deep.

Nutritional Values (per piece)			
Calories:	72.1	Fiber:	.712 g
Carbohydrates:	11.9 g	Protein:	1.51 g
Cholesterol:	8.88 mg	Sodium:	19.8 mg
Fat:	2.17 g		

Cookies

Banana Cookies

1 cup sugar substitute
½ cup diet margarine
⅓ cup mashed ripe banana
1 teaspoon vanilla extract
1 egg
2¼ cups flour
1 teaspoon baking soda
⅛ teaspoon ground nutmeg
1½ cups low fat granola

Preheat oven to 325° F. In a large bowl, cream the sugar substitute and diet margarine until fluffy. Add the mashed banana, vanilla extract and the egg. Beat well. In a small bowl place the flour, baking soda and nutmeg. Mix well with a fork. Add the dry mixture to the creamed mixture in the large bowl. Mix well. Drop by teaspoons onto a nonstick cookie sheet. Bake for 10 to 12 minutes. Remove cookies immediately from the cookie sheet to a wire rack to cool. Cookies will be 1" diameter. Yield: 72 cookies.

Nutritional Values (per piece)

Calories:	29.2	Fiber:	.275 g
Carbohydrates:	4.82 g	Protein:	.698 g
Cholesterol:	2.96 mg	Sodium:	10.3 mg
Fat:	.851 g		

Carob Chip Cookies

2¼ cups flour
1 teaspoon baking soda
¼ teaspoon salt substitute
½ cup sugar substitute
¾ cup brown sugar substitute
½ cup diet margarine
2 large eggs
1 teaspoon vanilla extract
2½ cups carob chips

Preheat oven to 375° F. In a large bowl, mix together the flour, baking soda, salt substitute, sugar substitute and brown sugar substitute. Add the margarine and blend well. Add the eggs and vanilla extract. Beat well. Add the carob chips and mix well. Drop by 1" diameter spoonfuls onto an ungreased baking sheet. Bake 7 to 10 minutes. Yield: 72 cookies.

Nutritional Values (per piece)

Calories:	59	Fiber:	1.28 g
Carbohydrates:	7.33 g	Protein:	1.76 g
Cholesterol:	6.55 mg	Sodium:	7.38 mg
Fat:	2.52 g		

Oatmeal Cookies

1 cup polyunsaturated oil
¾ cup granulated sugar substitute
1 cup firmly packed brown sugar substitute
2 large eggs
1 teaspoon vanilla extract
2 cups flour
1 teaspoon baking soda
½ teaspoon baking powder
½ teaspoon salt substitute
2 cups uncooked oatmeal
1 cup shredded coconut

Preheat oven to 350° F. Place the oil, granulated sugar substitute and imitation brown sugar in a bowl. Beat well. Add eggs and vanilla extract. Mix well. Add the flour, baking soda, baking powder and salt substitute to the beaten mixture a little at a time. Mix well with each addition of ingredients. Add the oats and coconut. Mix well. Shape into 1" diameter balls. Place on a cookie sheet. With a fork, flatten each ball, leaving the fork prong imprints in the flattened ball. Place in the oven and bake 5 to 7 minutes. Yield: 84 cookies.

Nutritional Values (per piece)

Calories:	45.8		Fiber:	3.52 g
Carbohydrates:	3.29 g		Protein:	.665 g
Cholesterol:	5.07 mg		Sodium:	18 mg
Fat:	3.4 g			

Carob and Coconut Macaroons

1 cup carob chips
2 large egg whites
¼ teaspoon cream of tartar
⅓ cup sugar substitute
1 teaspoon vanilla extract
2½ cups grated coconut

Preheat oven to 375° F. Place the carob chips in the top of a double boiler. Melt carob chips. While carob chips are melting, place the egg whites and cream of tartar in a large bowl. Beat the egg whites and cream of tartar until it holds stiff peaks. Fold in the melted carob chips, sugar substitute, and vanilla extract. Add the grated coconut. Place by teaspoonfuls on a nonstick cookie sheet. Bake for 20 minutes. Remove from oven and place on a wire rack to cool. Yield: 40 1" diameter macaroons.

Nutritional Values (per piece)

Calories:	56.1	Fiber:	.838 g
Carbohydrates:	3.56 g	Protein:	1.28 g
Cholesterol:	11 mg	Sodium:	4.97 mg
Fat:	4.33 g		

@

Cherry Coconut Macaroons

2 large egg whites
$1/4$ teaspoon cream of tartar
$1/3$ cup sugar substitute
1 teaspoon almond extract
$2^1/4$ cups grated coconut

Preheat oven to 375° F. Place the egg whites and cream of tartar in a large bowl. Beat until stiff peaks form. Continue beating, adding the sugar substitute. Fold in the almond extract. Then fold in the grated coconut. Mixture will be stiff. Drop by teaspoonsful onto a nonstick cookie sheet. Bake 20 minutes. Remove macaroons to a wire rack to cool. Cookies will be 1" in diameter. Yield: 35 pieces.

Nutritional Values (per piece)

Calories:	34.1	Fiber:	.826 g
Carbohydrates:	1.26 g	Protein:	.546 g
Cholesterol:	0 mg	Sodium:	5 mg
Fat:	3.23 g		

Lemon Biscotti

3½ cups flour
1 tablespoon baking powder
½ cup margarine
½ cup sugar substitute
5 eggs
2 tablespoons freshly grated lemon peel
1 teaspoon vanilla extract
1 cup pine nuts
¾ cup pistachio nuts
1 egg white, lightly beaten
¾ teaspoon powdered Isomalt®

In a large bowl, combine the flour and baking powder. In another large bowl, combine the margarine and sugar substitute. Beat until fluffy and light in color. Add the 5 eggs, lemon peel and vanilla extract. Beat until mixture is smooth and thick. Add the flour gradually. Mix well after each addition. Add the pine nuts and the pistachio nuts. Blend well. Gather the dough into a ball. Divide the dough into 3 equal parts. Wrap each part in plastic wrap. Refrigerate for 5 hours.

Preheat the oven to 350° F. Use a nonstick baking sheet or lightly grease a baking sheet with low-calorie cooking spray.

Remove the dough from the refrigerator. Transfer each section to a lightly floured surface. Shape each portion into a large log. Place 2 of the logs on 1 sheet about 5 inches apart. Place the remaining log on another cooking sheet. Brush each log with the egg white. Sprinkle with ¼ teaspoon powdered Isomalt® on each log.

Place the logs in the oven. Bake 30 to 35 minutes or until the dough has flattened somewhat and the top is slightly cracked. Remove from the oven. Using a large metal spatula, loosen the dough from the sheet. Leave on the sheet for 10 minutes. Carefully transfer the logs, one at a time, to a cutting board.

With a large knife, slice each log into diagonal slices that are 3" long by ¼" thick. Return the sliced biscotti to the baking sheets.

Bake for 10 to 15 minutes, turning twice, until the biscotti are dry and lightly toasted. Remove from oven and cool on racks. Yield: 60 pieces.

Nutritional Yield (per peice)

Calories:	69.3	Fiber:	.836 g
Carbohydrates:	6.88 g	Protein:	2.03 g
Cholesterol:	13.1 mg	Sodium:	15.4 mg
Fat:	4.2 g		

Vanilla Drops

1 cup margarine
½ cup powdered Isomalt®
1 teaspoon vanilla extract
2 cups flour

In a large bowl, cream the margarine until light and fluffy. Add the powdered Isomalt® and vanilla extract. Beat well. Add the flour a little at a time. Mix well. Cover the bowl and place in the refrigerator for 30 minutes.

Preheat the oven to 375° F. Remove the dough from the refrigerator. Shape into 1" balls. Place 1" apart on an ungreased baking sheet. Bake 12 minutes. Cookies will be a light golden color. Place the cookies on a cooling rack.

While cookies are in the oven, powder ¼ cup Isomalt®. When cookies are on the cooling rack, dust each cookie with the powdered Isomalt®. Let cool. Yield: 60 cookies.

Nutritional Values (per piece)

Calories:	28.4	Fiber:	.136 g
Carbohydrates:	3.2 g	Protein:	.449 g
Cholesterol:	0	Sodium:	13.4 mg
Fat:	1.51 g		

Lemon Squares

1 cup margarine
½ cup sugar substitute
½ teaspoon salt substitute
1 egg
1 egg yolk
2 tablespoons fresh lemon juice
1 teaspoon vanilla extract
4 cups floor

Combine the margarine, sugar substitute and salt substitute together in a large bowl. Beat until light and fluffy. Add the egg, the egg yolk, lemon juice and vanilla extract. Beat until well blended. Then gradually add the flour. Beat until mixed.

Remove the dough from the bowl and form into 2 large balls. Wrap each large ball in plastic wrap. Place the wrapped balls in the refrigerator for 4 hours.

Preheat oven to 350° F. Use a greased baking sheet or a baking sheet with a nonstick surface.

Remove the dough from the refrigerator. On a lightly floured surface roll out each ball to ⅛ inch thickness. Using a sharp knife cut into 1" squares or use cookie cutters of this size. Place each cookie on the baking sheet 1" apart. Bake for 10 minutes. The edges should be a light brown. Remove from oven and place on racks to cool. Yield: 80 cookies.

Nutritional Values (per piece)

Calories:	33.4		Fiber:	.206 g
Carbohydrates:	4.82 g		Protein:	.719 g
Cholesterol:	1.96 mg		Sodium:	10.7 mg
Fat:	1.21 g			

Peanut Butter Cookies

2 cups smooth dietetic peanut butter
1 cup sugar substitute
2 eggs
60 carob chips

Preheat the oven to 350° F. In a bowl, combine the peanut butter, sugar substitute and eggs. Blend thoroughly. Flour your hands and form the mixture into 2" diameter balls. Place the balls on an ungreased baking sheet. Make sure there are at least 2 inches between the balls. The cookies need plenty of room to spread. Then place a carob chip in the center of each cookie. Place in the oven and bake for 12 minutes. Remove from the oven and place on a cooling rack. Yield: 60 cookies.

Nutritional Values (per piece)

Calories:	53.1	Fiber:	.563 g
Carbohydrates:	1.97 g	Protein:	2.26 g
Cholesterol:	6.25 mg	Sodium:	2.36 mg
Fat:	4.43 g		

Heavenly Puffs

1 cup margarine
1 cup sugar substitute
2 eggs
2¾ cups flour
2 teaspoons cream of tartar
1 teaspoon baking soda
¼ teaspoon salt substitute
2 teaspoons ground cinnamon
¼ teaspoon sugar substitute

Place the margarine, 1 cup sugar substitute and eggs in a large bowl. Beat well. Mixture will be light and fluffy.

In a medium sized bowl combine the flour, cream of tartar, baking soda and salt substitute. Mix well. Add this mixture to the light and fluffy mixture in the large bowl. Blend well. Cover the large bowl and place in the refrigerator for an hour.

Remove bowl from refrigerator. Preheat the oven to 375° F. In a small bowl, mix the cinnamon plus ¼ teaspoon sugar substitute. Mix well. Shape the dough in the large bowl into balls 2" in diameter. Roll in the cinnamon and sugar mixture. Place the balls 3" apart on an ungreased baking sheet. Bake the cookies 12 to 15 minutes (until golden brown). Yield: 35 cookies.

Nutritional Values (per piece)

Calories:	102	Fiber:	.743 g
Carbohydrates:	16 g	Protein:	2.51 g
Cholesterol:	12.2 mg	Sodium:	62.9 mg
Fat:	3.01 g		

Pies

Pie Crust

1 cup flour
1 teaspoon sugar substitute
¼ teaspoon salt substitute
3 tablespoons vegetable shortening
3 tablespoons ice water

In a bowl, combine the flour, sugar substitute and salt substitute. Add the vegetable shortening and cut with 2 knives or pastry cutter. Add the ice water and knead until well mixed. If needed, more ice water can be added. Place on a floured board. Roll out to desired thickness. Yield: 1 pie crust (10 slices).

Nutritional Values (per slice)

Calories:	68.2	Fiber:	.409 g
Carbohydrates:	9.54 g	Protein:	1.29 g
Cholesterol:	0 mg	Sodium:	.25 mg
Fat:	2.69 g		

⊙

Graham Cracker Crust

1 cup finely crushed graham crackers
¼ cup melted diet margarine

Preheat oven to 350° F. Combine the crushed graham crackers and melted diet margarine in a bowl. Mix well. Press into the bottom and on the sides of a 9" pie pan. Bake 8 to 10 minutes. Yield: 1 pie crust (10 slices).

Nutritional Values (per slice)

Calories:	70.4	Fiber:	.324 g
Carbohydrates:	9.24 g	Protein:	.856 g
Cholesterol:	0 mg	Sodium:	92.6 mg
Fat:	3.41 g		

Pumpkin Pie

1 Pie Crust (page 117)
1 large can pumpkin
1 cup evaporated milk
1 teaspoon pumpkin pie spice
1 teaspoon vanilla extract
3 egg yolks
10 teaspoons frozen diet whipped topping

Preheat oven to 350° F. Prepare pie crust. Place rolled out crust in the bottom of a 9" pie pan. Flute edges of crust. In a large bowl, place the pumpkin, evaporated milk, pumpkin pie spice, vanilla extract and egg yolks. Beat well with a wooden spoon. Continue beating until well mixed. Then pour into pie shell. Sprinkle top with nutmeg. Bake 40 to 45 minutes. Place on a wire rack to cool. Then refrigerate. Cut into 10 wedges. Place 1 teaspoon of diet frozen whipped topping on each piece just before serving. Yield: 10 pieces.

Nutritional Values (per serving)

Calories:	58.1	Fiber:	1.27 g
Carbohydrates:	7.03 g	Protein:	3.29 g
Cholesterol:	64.8 mg	Sodium:	34.1 mg
Fat:	2.11 g		

Apple Pie

2 Pie Crusts (page 117)
8 cooking apples, peeled, cored and sliced
1 tablespoon lemon juice
2 tablespoons flour
1 teaspoon cinnamon
½ teaspoon nutmeg
⅛ teaspoon ginger

Preheat oven to 350° F. In a large bowl place the peeled, cored and sliced apples. Add lemon juice, flour, cinnamon, nutmeg and ginger. Mix well. Roll out the pie crust. Place the pie crust in a 9" pie pan. Add the apple mixture. Roll out another pie crust and place on top of apple mixture. Slice to release steam. Flute edges. Bake 40 minutes. Can be served warm or when cooled. Yield: 10 pieces.

Nutritional Values (per serving)

Calories:	71.2	Fiber:	2.23 g
Carbohydrates:	18.2 g	Protein:	.377 g
Cholesterol:	0 mg	Sodium:	.047 mg
Fat:	.415 g		

9

Peach Pie

2 Pie Crusts (page 117)
5 cups sliced fresh peaches
¼ cup flour
1 teaspoon lemon juice
1 teaspoon cinnamon
1 teaspoon allspice
10 teaspoons diet frozen whipped topping

Preheat oven to 425° F. In a bowl, mix together the peaches, flour, lemon juice, cinnamon and allspice. Place a rolled out pie crust in a 9" pie pan. Roll out a second piece for the top of the pie. Place the peach mixture in the pie pan on top of the crust. Place the second piece of rolled out pie crust on top of peach mixture. Cut a design for steam to be released. Flute the edges. Bake at 425° F for 15 minutes. Then reduce the heat to 350° F, and continue to bake for 25 minutes. Cool. Cut into 10 2" wedges. Place 1 teaspoon of diet frozen whipped topping on each wedge. Serve immediately. Yield: 10 pieces.

Nutritional Values (per serving)

Calories:	52		Fiber:	1.63 g
Carbohydrates:	12.2 g		Protein:	.935 g
Cholesterol:	0 mg		Sodium:	.384 mg
Fat:	.425 g			

Pineapple Pie

1 Graham Cracker Crust (page 118)
1 package (1 ounce) sugar-free instant vanilla pud-
  ding mix
1 cup diet sour cream
1 cup dietetic canned crushed pineapple, drained
½ teaspoon sugar substitute

Prepare graham cracker crust. Place crust in a 9" pie pan. In a bowl, combine the pudding mix and sour cream. Beat well until completely blended. Add the pineapple. Stir well. Add the sugar substitute. Stir until well blended. Pour into the prepared graham cracker crust. Refrigerate for 4 hours before serving. Yield: 10 pieces.

Nutritional Values (per serving)			
Calories:	92.8	Fiber:	.512 g
Carbohydrates:	12.4 g	Protein:	1.69 g
Cholesterol:	9.44 mg	Sodium:	87.7 mg
Fat:	4.21 g		

Avocado Pie

Pie crust

¾ cup fat-free graham cracker crumbs
¾ teaspoon sugar substitute
4 egg whites

Place graham cracker crumbs, sugar substitute and egg whites in a blender. Process until the mixture is moist and crumbly. Place mixture in an 8" pie pan. Press mixture into the bottom of the pan and up the sides.

Filling

¼ cup hot water
1 package Knox gelatin
2 medium sized avocados
1 can condensed milk
2 tablespoons lemon juice
1 cup diet whipped topping

In a small bowl, place the hot water and Knox gelatin. Set aside. Place the avocados, condensed milk, lemon juice and Knox gelatin mixture in a blender. Blend until well mixed. Pour into pie crust. Spread the dairy topping over the top. Refrigerate for 2 hours. Yield: 8 wedges.

Nutritional Values (per serving)

Calories:	238	Fiber:	2.08 g
Carbohydrates:	27 g	Protein:	4.91 g
Cholesterol:	13 mg	Sodium:	57.8 mg
Fat:	13.4 g		

Hodge Podge

Raspberry Crunch

½ cup fresh raspberries, crushed
1 cup margarine
1 cup sugar substitute
2 teaspoons vanilla extract
2 egg yolks
2½ cups sifted flour
1 cup chopped pecans

Place the raspberries in a blender. Blend at low speed until raspberries are crushed but not liquid. Place the margarine, sugar substitute, vanilla and egg yolks in a bowl. Beat at high speed until light and fluffy. Gradually stir in the flour as you continue to beat. When completely blended, shape into a ball and place in a plastic bag or plastic wrap. Put in the refrigerator and leave for 4 hours.

Preheat the oven to 300° F. Remove the dough from the refrigerator. Shape the dough into 1" balls. Place the balls on a cookie sheet 1½" apart. Using a wooden spoon, make an indentation in the center of each cookie. Fill each cookie with 1 teaspoon of fresh, crushed raspberries. Bake the cookies for 20 minutes. Remove to cooling racks. Yield: 48 cookies.

Nutritional Values (per piece)

Calories:	55.9	Fiber:	.339 g
Carbohydrates:	5.24 g	Protein:	1.06 g
Cholesterol:	8.88 mg	Sodium:	20 mg
Fat:	3.45 g		

🌀

Sweet Snack

3 cups presweetened carob chips
1 cup banana chips
1 cup raisins
1 cup chopped English walnuts
1 cup chopped peanuts

Place the presweetened carob chips in the top of a double boiler and melt. Add the banana chips, raisins, English walnuts and peanuts. Mix well. Drop by 1" balls onto waxed paper. Place in the refrigerator to cool. Yield: 60 1" snacks.

Nutritional Values (per piece)

Calories:	60.2	Fiber:	.461 mg
Carbohydrates:	5.78 g	Protein:	1.54 g
Cholesterol:	.302 mg	Sodium:	.728 mg
Fat:	3.81 g		

☻

Trail Mix

20 unsalted low fat saltine crackers
1 cup raisins
1 cup peanuts
2 cups presweetened carob chips

In a medium sized bowl, crumble the saltine crackers into bite sized pieces. Add the raisins, peanuts and carob chips. Mix well. Place in the refrigerator. Measure ½ cup each and place in plastic sandwich sized bags. Yield: 65 servings.

Nutritional Values (per serving)

Calories:	30.6		Fiber:	.274 g
Carbohydrates:	3.83 g		Protein:	.876 g
Cholesterol:	.07 mg		Sodium:	10.2 mg
Fat:	1.5 g			

Spice Delight

4 cups flour
1 teaspoon ground cinnamon
1 teaspoon ground nutmeg
1/2 teaspoon ground ginger
1/4 teaspoon ground cloves
1 1/2 cups margarine
1/2 cup sugar substitute
1 egg
1 teaspoon vanilla extract

In a large bowl, combine the flour, cinnamon, nutmeg, ginger, and cloves. In another large bowl, beat the margarine and sugar substitute together until light and fluffy. Add the egg and the vanilla extract. Beat until well blended. Then with the mixer on low speed, gradually add the flour and spice mixture. Mix until well blended.

Separate the dough into 3 equal parts. Flatten each piece to 1" thick. Wrap in plastic wrap and refrigerate for 1 hour.

Preheat oven to 375° F. Remove the dough from the refrigerator. On a lightly floured surface, roll out each of the 3 sections, 1 section at a time, to 1/4" thick. Use a cookie cutter for fun shapes or a sharp knife and cut into 1" squares. Place the cookies 1" apart on an ungreased baking sheet. Bake for 10 minutes or until the edges are lightly browned. Place cookies on a rack to cool. Yield: 80 cookies.

Nutritional Values (per piece)

Calories:	38.5	Fiber:	.23 g
Carbohydrates:	4.84 g	Protein:	.728 g
Cholesterol:	1.96 mg	Sodium:	15.7 mg
Fat:	1.77 g		

9

Chocolate Bars

1 cup firmly packed brown sugar substitute
1 cup diet margarine
1 egg yolk
1 teaspoon vanilla extract
2 cups flour
⅛ teaspoon salt substitute
2 cups melted carob
1 cup finely chopped walnuts

Preheat oven to 350°. In a large mixing bowl, cream the brown sugar substitute and the diet margarine together. Add the egg yolk, vanilla extract, flour and salt substitute. Mix well. Spread mixture in a 9" x 13" nonstick pan. Bake 20 to 25 minutes. While bars are baking, melt carob in the top of a double boiler. When bars are removed from the oven, pour the melted carob over the bars. Then sprinkle the chopped walnuts on top of the carob bars. Let cool completely. Cut into 2" long x 1" wide bars. Bars will be 1" thick. Yield: 72 bars.

Nutritional Values (per piece)

Calories:	54.2		Fiber:	.114 g
Carbohydrates:	6.12 g		Protein:	1.35 g
Cholesterol:	3.46 mg		Sodium:	11.3 mg
Fat:	2.72 g			

Maple Bars

1 cup packed brown sugar substitute
⅓ cup diet margarine
1½ teaspoon maple extract
1 teaspoon vanilla extract
1 egg
1 egg white
2 cups flour
¾ teaspoon baking soda
½ teaspoon ground cinnamon
¼ teaspoon ground allspice

Preheat oven to 325° F. In a small bowl, combine the brown sugar substitute and diet margarine. Beat until fluffy. Add the maple extract, vanilla extract, egg and egg white. Beat very well. In a large bowl, combine the flour, baking soda, cinnamon and allspice. Mix together with a fork. Add the ingredients from the small bowl to the large bowl, a little at a time. Stir well. Drop by teaspoons onto a nonstick cooking sheet. Shape into bars. Place in the oven and bake 8 to 10 minutes. Cookies will be 1" long x ¼" wide x ¼" deep. Yield: 72 bars.

Nutritional Values (per piece)

Calories:	17.3	Fiber:	.114 g
Carbohydrates:	2.66 g	Protein:	.45 g
Cholesterol:	2.96 mg	Sodium:	17.8 mg
Fat:	.512 g		

🌀

Brownies

1 cup sugar substitute
¼ cup polyunsaturated oil
¼ cup plain nonfat yogurt
1 teaspoon vanilla extract
3 egg whites
½ cup flour
½ cup powdered carob
¼ teaspoon baking powder
⅛ teaspoon salt substitute
¼ cup carob chips

Preheat oven to 375° F. In a large bowl, combine the sugar substitute, oil, yogurt, vanilla extract and egg whites. Mix well. Set aside. In another bowl combine the flour, powdered carob, baking powder and salt substitute. Mix well. Add this mixture to the mixture in the large bowl. Mix until well moistened. Place the mixture in a 9" square nonstick cake pan. Bake for 25 minutes. Remove from the oven and sprinkle the top with ¼ cup carob chips. Let stand until the carob chips begin to melt. Spread over the top of the brownies with a spatula. Cool. Yield: 36 1" square brownies.

Nutritional Values (per piece)

Calories:	38.2	Fiber:	.626 g
Carbohydrates:	4.03 g	Protein:	.852 g
Cholesterol:	.292 mg	Sodium:	4.32 mg
Fat:	2.09 g		

Fruit Crêpes

2 eggs, beaten
1 cup whole milk
1 cup flour
4 sliced, cored and peeled apples
¼ teaspoon cinnamon
1 teaspoon polyunsaturated oil

Place the eggs in a medium sized bowl and beat well. Add the milk and flour. Mix well. Cover the bowl and allow to stand at room temperature for 30 minutes. Prepare the apples by slicing, coring and peeling. Add cinnamon to prepared apples. Stir well to coat the sliced apples. Heat and add 1 teaspoon polyunsaturated oil to a 6" frying pan (or use a nonstick crêpe pan). Pour batter to cover bottom of pan. When light brown, turn and brown the other side. Remove from heat. Add 1 tablespoon prepared apples to half of the cooked crêpe. Fold top over the apples and place on serving plate. Yield: 12 crêpes.

Nutritional Values (per serving)

Calories:	58.3		Fiber:	.907 g
Carbohydrates:	8.14 g		Protein:	2.32 g
Cholesterol:	56 mg		Sodium:	25.8 mg
Fat:	2.1 g			

@

Prune Purée

¼ cup diet maple syrup
2 tablespoons sugar substitute
1 12-ounce package whole, pitted prunes
⅔ cup water

In a food blender, place the diet maple syrup, sugar substitute and the prunes. Blend well. Slowly add the water. Blend until mixture is smooth. Purée can be used in recipes noted in this cookbook or use on toast for a special treat. Yield: 2 cups.

Nutritional Values (2 cups)			
Calories:	454	Fiber:	15.7 g
Carbohydrates:	119 g	Protein:	4.45 g
Cholesterol:	0 mg	Sodium:	63.5 mg
Fat:	.885 g		

Chocolate Soufflé

5 tablespoons sugar substitute
½ cup Prune Purée (page 135)
2 ounces sweetened carob, grated
6 egg whites
¼ teaspoon cream of tartar
⅛ teaspoon salt substitute

Coat a 1½ quart soufflé pan with diet cooking spray. Sprinkle with 1 tablespoon sugar substitute and set aside. Preheat oven to 350° F. In a medium bowl, combine 2 tablespoons sugar substitute, Prune Purée and grated carob. Set aside. In another bowl, beat the egg whites, cream of tartar and salt substitute until soft peaks form. Gradually add the remaining 2 tablespoons sugar substitute and beat until stiff peaks form. Fold the egg white mixture into the Prune Purée mixture. Spoon the mixture into the soufflé pan. Place the soufflé pan in a 9" x 9" square baking pan. Add hot water to the pan to 1" depth. Gently place in the preheated oven and bake for 55 minutes. If you desire, sprinkle the top with ⅛ teaspoon sugar substitute. Serve immediately. Yield: 12 2-ounce servings.

Nutritional Values (per serving)

Calories:	40.2	Fiber:	1.54 g
Carbohydrates:	10.3 g	Progein:	.333 g
Cholesterol:	0 mg	Sodium:	5.26 mg
Fat:	.059 g		

Custard Tarts

1 cup flour
⅓ cup unsalted margarine
4 tablespoons unsweetened apple juice
¾ cup sugar-free applesauce
½ cup whole milk
2 eggs
½ teaspoon cinnamon
1 apple, sliced and cored

Preheat oven to 425° F. In a medium sized bowl, combine the flour and margarine. Add enough fruit juice to form a soft dough. Knead well. Pinch off small pieces and press into nonstick tart pans or small muffin tin wells. Set aside. In a blender, place the applesauce, milk, eggs and cinnamon. Blend well. Fill each tart ¾ full. Sprinkle tops with cinnamon. Bake at 425° F for 10 minutes. Then reduce heat to 350° F. Continue baking another 20 to 25 minutes. Place on wire rack to cool. Refrigerate 1 hour. When ready to serve, place one apple slice on top of each tart. Yield: 20 tarts.

Nutritional Values (per serving)

Calories:	56.9	Fiber:	.355 g
Carbohydrates:	7.63 g	Protein:	1.52 g
Cholesterol:	22.1 mg	Sodium:	23.6 mg
Fat:	2.27 g		

❾

Peach Tarts

1 cup flour
⅓ cup diet margarine
4 tablespoons unsweetened apple juice
2¼ cups chopped fresh peaches
3 tablespoons corn starch

Preheat oven to 375° F. In a medium sized bowl, mix together the flour, diet margarine and unsweetened apple juice. Knead well. Break off small pieces and press into nonstick tart pans or small muffin tin wells. Place the peaches and cornstarch in a belnder and blend well. Then pour into the top of a double boiler. Heat over medium heat, stirring constantly until mixture thickens. Remove from heat. Fill each tart half full. Bake for 20 to 25 minutes. Place on wire rack to cool. Sprinkle cooled tarts with cinnamon or nutmeg if you desire. Yield: 20 tarts.

Nutritional Values (per serving)			
Calories:	54.4	Fiber:	.574 g
Carbohydrates:	9.45 g	Protein:	.819 g
Cholesterol:	0 mg	Sodium:	14.4 mg
Fat:	1.56 g		

Pumpkin Tarts

1 Pie Crust (page 117)
1 cup unsweetened canned pumpkin
1 cup whole milk
½ cup sugar substitute
¾ teaspoon vanilla extract
½ teaspoon pumpkin pie spice
¼ teaspoon butter flavored extract
2 eggs, beaten lightly
2 egg whites, beaten lightly
⅓ cup nondairy whipped topping

Preheat oven to 350° F. Make the pie crust. Before rolling out, set aside. In a large bowl, combine the above ingredients. Mix very well. Set aside. Roll out the pie crust. Place in a 10" round nonstick tart pan. Prick the bottom of the crust with a fork in several places. Place the pumpkin mixture in the crust. Bake for 40 minutes. The filling will be almost set. Remove from oven. Cool at least 30 to 40 minutes. Spread the nondairy topping on the tart. Cut into wedges 1" across. Serve immediately. Yield: 40 tarts.

Nutritional Values (per serving)

Calories:	12.3	Fiber:	.172 g
Carbohydrates:	.973 g	Protein:	.75 g
Cholesterol:	11.5 g	Sodium:	9.11 mg
Fat:	.63 g		

〰️

Frozen Fruit

2 cans dietetic crushed pineapple, undrained
1 can dietetic cherry pie filling
1 can evaporated skim milk
1 8-ounce carton diet frozen whipped topping
  (thawed)
36 green or red maraschino cherries

In a large bowl, mix the dietetic crushed pineapple, dietetic cherry pie filling and evaporated skim milk. Fold in the diet frozen whipped topping. Blend well. Pour mixture into a 13" x 9" nonstick pan. Cover and place in the freezer at least 2 hours or until thoroughly frozen. When ready to serve, cut and place 1 maraschino cherry on each piece. Cut pieces 2" x 2" square. Yield: 36 pieces.

Nutritional Values (per piece)

Calories:	41		Fiber:	.254 g
Carbohydrates:	6.01 g		Protein:	.79 g
Cholesterol:	.283 mg		Sodium:	11.5 mg
Fat:	1.75 g			

@

Haupia
(Hawaiian Sweet Treat)

3 packages Knox gelatin
½ cup water
1 can coconut milk
⅔ cup sugar substitute
1 cup skim milk

Combine the 3 packages of Knox gelatin and ½ cup water. Set aside. In a heavy pot, combine the coconut milk and sugar substitute. Heat until the sugar substitute dissolves. Do not boil. Add the gelatin mixture. Stir well. Remove from heat. Add the skim milk. Mix well. Allow mixture to cool. Stir the mixture again as it begins to gel. Then pour into an 8" x 8" square pan. Refrigerate. Cut into 2" squares. Mixture will be 2" square x 1" thick. Yield: 80 pieces.

Nutritional Values (per piece)

Calories:	7.51		Fiber:	.032 g
Carbohydrates:	.228 g		Protein:	.387 g
Cholesterol:	.055 mg		Sodium:	2.46 mg
Fat:	.607 g			

Maple Pudding

1 package sugar-free maple pudding and pie filling
  mix
1 8-ounce carton plain low fat yogurt
1 8-ounce carton vanilla low fat yogurt
1 cup chopped English walnuts
½ cup diet frozen whipped topping (thawed)

In a large bowl, place the maple pudding mix, plain low fat yogurt, vanilla low fat yogurt and chopped English walnuts. Mix well. Fold in the thawed frozen whipped topping. Spoon ½ cup each into serving bowls. Refrigerate 3 hours before serving. If desired, sprinkle top with a dash of ground cinnamon. Yield: 12 servings.

Nutritional Values (per serving)

Calories:	100	Fiber:	.456 g
Carbohydrates:	6.15 g	Protein:	3.98 g
Cholesterol:	1.05 mg	Sodium:	41.7 mg
Fat:	7.15 g		

⊙

Bread Pudding

2 cups low fat milk
1 cup egg substitute
¾ cup Prune Purée (page 135)
¾ cup sugar substitute
½ cup evaporated skim milk
2 tablespoons diet margarine, melted
1 teaspoon vanilla extract
⅓ cup carob powder
6 French bread slices (cut ¾ inch thick and one
    inch square)
1 teaspoon powdered cinnamon

In a large bowl, combine the low fat milk, egg substitute, Prune Purée, sugar substitute, evaporated skim milk, margarine, vanilla extract and carob powder. Blend very well. Add the bread cubes and mix. Place the mixture in 8 8-ounce pudding cups. Cover and place in the refrigerator for 3 hours.

Preheat oven to 350° F. Uncover the pudding cups. Bake for 45 minutes. Sprinkle the tops with cinnamon. Serve immediately. Yield: 8 servings.

Nutritional Values (per serving)

Calories:	161	Fiber:	2.44 g
Carbohydrates:	22.5 g	Protein:	9.59 g
Cholesterol:	1.99 mg	Sodium:	279 mg
Fat:	3.38 g		

Cherry Scones

¾ cup dried cherries
¼ cup boiling water
1¾ cup flour
½ cup sugar substitute
¼ cup yellow cornmeal
2 teaspoons baking powder
⅛ teaspoon salt substitute
2 tablespoons diet margarine
⅓ cup plain nonfat yogurt
¼ cup evaporated skim milk
1 teaspoon vanilla extract
½ teaspoon imitation butter extract
1 egg white, beaten lightly
3 teaspoons sugar substitute

Preheat oven to 425° F. In a bowl, place the cherries and the boiling water. Set aside. In a large bowl, mix the flour, ½ cup sugar substitute, cornmeal, baking powder and salt substitute. Cut in the diet margarine with two knives or a pastry blender. Mixture will be coarse. Drain the water off the softened cherries. Blend in the bowl with the cherries the yogurt, skim milk and extracts. Add the blended ingredients, a little at a time, to the dry ingredients mixed in the large bowl. Stir just until the dry ingredients are moist. The dough will be sticky. Place the sticky dough in an 8" x 8" square nonstick cake pan. Brush the beaten egg white over the top of the dough. Sprinkle the top of the egg whites with the 3 teaspoons sugar substitute. Bake in the oven for 20 minutes. Remove from oven. Can be served warm or when cooled. Yield: 16 scones.

Nutritional Values (per piece)

Calories:	110		Fiber:	1.05 g
Carbohydrates:	21.1 g		Protein:	2.75 g
Cholesterol:	.56 mg		Sodium:	21.8 mg
Fat:	2.73 g			

Appendix: Complete Nutritional Values

⊚ After Dinner Mints

Calories	1.56	Pantothenic	.008 mg
Protein	.084 g	Vitamin C	.024 mg
Carbohydrates	.119 g	Vitamin D	.025 mcg
Fat—Total	.085 g	Vitamin E-Alpha E	.002 mg
Saturated Fat	.053 g	Calcium	3.02 mg
Monounsaturated Fat	.024 g	Copper	0 mg
Polyunsaturated Fat	.003 g	Iron	.001 mg
Omega 3 Fatty Acid	.001 g	Magnesium	.341 mg
Omega 6 Fatty Acid	.002 g	Manganese	0 mg
Cholesterol	.346 mg	Phosphorus	2.38 mg
Dietary Fiber	0 g	Potassium	3.86 mg
Total Vitamin A	.788 RE	Selenium	.051 mcg
A–Retinol	.686 RE	Sodium	1.25 mg
A–Carotenoi	.076 RE	Zinc	.01 mg
Thiamin–B1	.001 mg	Complex Carbohydrates	0 g
Riboflavin–B2	.004 mg	Sugars	.119 g
Niacin–B3	.002 mg	Mono-Saccharide	0 g
Niacin Equivalent	.002 mg	Di-Saccharide	.119 g
Vitamin B6	.001 mg	Alcohol	0 g
Vitamin B12	.009 mcg	Caffeine	0 mg
Folate	.127 mcg	Water	2.24 g

⊚ Almond Balls

Calories	72.2	Pantothenic	.132 mg
Protein	2.08 g	Vitamin C	.893 mg
Carbohydrates	9.62 g	Vitamin D	.054 mcg
Fat—Total	2.9 g	Vitamin E-Alpha E	.591 mg
Saturated Fat	1.1 g	Calcium	37.5 mg
Monounsaturated Fat	1.06 g	Copper	.045 mg
Polyunsaturated	.5 g	Iron	.526 mg
Omega 3 Fatty Acid	.015 g	Magnesium	9.45 mg
Omega 6 Fatty Acid	.484 g	Manganese	.128 mg
Cholesterol	7.63 mg	Phosphorus	27.4 mg
Dietary Fiber	.631 g	Potassium	71.3 mg
Total Vitamin A	14.4 RE	Selenium	2.85 mcg
A–Retinol	13.1 RE	Sodium	4.61 mg
A–Carotenoid	.97 RE	Zinc	.163 mg
Thiamin–B1	.067 mg	Complex Carbohydrates	6.35 g
Riboflavin–B2	.065 mg	Sugars	1.81 g
Niacin–B3	.606 mg	Mono-Saccharide	.075 g
Niacin Equivalent	.603 mg	Di-Saccharide	.267 g
Vitamin B6	.04 mg	Alcohol	0 g
Vitamin B12	.028 mcg	Caffeine	0 mg
Folate	6.69 mcg	Water	13.5 g

☺ Almond Delight

Calories	28.9	Pantothenic	.024 mg
Protein	1.09 g	Vitamin C	.072 mg
Carbohydrates	.909 g	Vitamin D	0 mcg
Fat—Total	2.54 g	Vitamin E-Alpha E	.271 mg
Saturated Fat	.241 g	Calcium	12 mg
Monounsaturated Fat	1.65 g	Copper	.052 mg
Polyunsaturated Fat	.533 g	Iron	.177 mg
Omega 3 Fatty Acid	.018 g	Magnesium	13.9 mg
Omega 6 Fatty Acid	.513 g	Manganese	.07 mg
Cholesterol	0 mg	Phosphorus	25.8 mg
Dietary Fiber	.474 g	Potassium	37.7 mg
Total Vitamin A	.002 RE	Selenium	.408 mcg
A–Retinol	0 RE	Sodium	2.15 mg
A–Carotenoi	.002 RE	Zinc	.154 mg
Thiamin–B1	.008 mg	Complex Carbohydrates	.156 g
Riboflavin–B2	.037 mg	Sugars	.281 g
Niacin–B3	.154 mg	Mono-Saccharide	.011 g
Niacin Equivalent	.155 mg	Di-Saccharide	0 g
Vitamin B6	.005 mg	Alcohol	0 g
Vitamin B12	.002 mcg	Caffeine	0 mg
Folate	1.9 mcg	Water	1.18 g

☺ Almond Pound Cake

Calories	56.8	Pantothenic	.098 mg
Protein	1.95 g	Vitamin C	.043 mg
Carbohydrates	8.82 g	Vitamin D	.375 mcg
Fat—Total	1.47 g	Vitamin E-Alpha E	.239 mg
Saturated Fat	.281 g	Calcium	27.2 mg
Monounsaturated Fat	.519 g	Copper	.017 mg
Polyunsaturated Fat	.541 g	Iron	.582 mg
Omega 3 Fatty Acid	.01 g	Magnesium	3.66 mg
Omega 6 Fatty Acid	.533 g	Manganese	.077 mg
Cholesterol	10.7 mg	Phosphorus	50.7 mg
Dietary Fiber	.358 g	Potassium	70.4 mg
Total Vitamin A	35.5 RE	Selenium	5.15 mcg
A–Retinol	33.1 RE	Sodium	21.3 mg
A–Carotenoi	2.32 RE	Zinc	.124 mg
Thiamin–B1	.089 mg	Complex Carbohydrates	8 g
Riboflavin–B2	.088 mg	Sugars	.463 g
Niacin–B3	.655 mg	Mono-Saccharide	.164 g
Niacin Equivalent	.655 mg	Di-Saccharide	.242 g
Vitamin B6	.01 mg	Alcohol	0 g
Vitamin B12	.049 mcg	Caffeine	0 mg
Folate	4.35 mcg	Water	11.5 g

☺ Apple Pie

Calories	71.2	Pantothenic	.076 mg
Protein	.377 g	Vitamin C	7 mg
Carbohydrates	18.2 g	Vitamin D	0 mcg
Fat—Total	.415 g	Vitamin E-Alpha E	.658 mg
Saturated Fat	.067 g	Calcium	8.07 mg
Monounsaturated Fat	.018 g	Copper	.048 mg
Polyunsaturated Fat	.124 g	Iron	.271 mg
Omega 3 Fatty Acid	.021 g	Magnesium	5.95 mg
Omega 6 Fatty Acid	.103 g	Manganese	.06 mg
Cholesterol	0 mg	Phosphorus	9.51 mg
Dietary Fiber	2.23 g	Potassium	131 mg
Total Vitamin A	5.88 RE	Selenium	.864 mcg
A–Retinol	0 RE	Sodium	.047 mg
A–Carotenoi	5.88 RE	Zinc	.056 mg
Thiamin–B1	.031 mg	Complex Carbohydrates	1.12 g
Riboflavin–B2	.023 mg	Sugars	13.4 g
Niacin–B3	.179 mg	Mono-Saccharide	9.25 g
Niacin Equivalent	.177 mg	Di-Saccharide	2.88 g
Vitamin B6	.054 mg	Alcohol	0 g
Vitamin B12	0 mcg	Caffeine	0 mg
Folate	3.69 mcg	Water	94.2 g

☺ Apple-Raisin Surprise

Calories	38.3	Pantothenic	.053 mg
Protein	.874 g	Vitamin C	.126 mg
Carbohydrates	3.38 g	Vitamin D	0 mcg
Fat—Total	2.65 g	Vitamin E-Alpha E	.549 mg
Saturated Fat	.717 g	Calcium	7.98 mg
Monounsaturated Fat	1.38 g	Copper	.082 mg
Polyunsaturated Fat	.425 g	Iron	.292 mg
Omega 3 Fatty Acid	.012 g	Magnesium	13.6 mg
Omega 6 Fatty Acid	.411 g	Manganese	.097 mg
Cholesterol	0 mg	Phosphorus	25.4 mg
Dietary Fiber	.487 g	Potassium	53.4 mg
Total Vitamin A	.051 RE	Selenium	.965 mcg
A–Retinol	0 RE	Sodium	1.55 mg
A–Carotenoi	.051 RE	Zinc	.213 mg
Thiamin–B1	.012 mg	Complex Carbohydrates	.631 g
Riboflavin–B2	.024 mg	Sugars	2.22 g
Niacin–B3	.136 mg	Mono-Saccharide	.443 g
Niacin Equivalent	.137 mg	Di-Saccharide	.582 g
Vitamin B6	.015 mg	Alcohol	0 g
Vitamin B12	0 mcg	Caffeine	0 mg
Folate	3.34 mcg	Water	2.36 g

⊚ Applesauce-Pineapple Cake

Calories	105	Pantothenic	.087 mg
Protein	1.27 g	Vitamin C	1.06 mg
Carbohydrates	9.58 g	Vitamin D	.755 mcg
Fat—Total	7.29 g	Vitamin E-Alpha E	.614 mg
Saturated Fat	.925 g	Calcium	19.1 mg
Monounsaturated Fat	2.26 g	Copper	.092 mg
Polyunsaturated Fat	3.75 g	Iron	.3 mg
Omega 3 Fatty Acid	.427 g	Magnesium	11.5 mg
Omega 6 Fatty Acid	3.3 g	Manganese	.267 mg
Cholesterol	.177 mg	Phosphorus	47.2 mg
Dietary Fiber	.544 g	Potassium	49.4 mg
Total Vitamin A	71.6 RE	Selenium	.355 mcg
A–Retinol	64.5 RE	Sodium	84 mg
A–Carotenoi	6.88 RE	Zinc	.185 mg
Thiamin–B1	.045 mg	Complex Carbohydrates	.949 g
Riboflavin–B2	.032 mg	Sugars	8.05 g
Niacin–B3	.254 mg	Mono-Saccharide	.242 g
Niacin Equivalent	.254 mg	Di-Saccharide	.268 g
Vitamin B6	.045 mg	Alcohol	0 g
Vitamin B12	0.15 mcg	Caffeine	0 mg
Folate	5.13 mcg	Water	16.7 g

⊚ Apricot Balls

Calories	10.8	Pantothenic	.024 mg
Protein	.175 g	Vitamin C	.908 mg
Carbohydrates	1.16 g	Vitamin D	.0 mcg
Fat—Total	.7 g	Vitamin E-Alpha E	.082 mg
Saturated Fat	.597 g	Calcium	1.36 mg
Monounsaturated Fat	.041 g	Copper	.016 mg
Polyunsaturated Fat	.013 g	Iron	.09 mg
Omega 3 Fatty Acid	0 g	Magnesium	1.26 mg
Omega 6 Fatty Acid	.013 g	Manganese	.036 mg
Cholesterol	0 mg	Phosphorus	3.73 mg
Dietary Fiber	.324 g	Potassium	29.9 mg
Total Vitamin A	19.8 RE	Selenium	.494 mcg
A–Retinol	0 RE	Sodium	.477 mg
A–Carotenoi	19.8 RE	Zinc	.042 mg
Thiamin–B1	.004 mg	Complex Carbohydrates	0 g
Riboflavin–B2	.003 mg	Sugars	.8 g
Niacin–B3	.057 mg	Mono-Saccharide	.252 g
Niacin Equivalent	.057 mg	Di-Saccharide	.478 g
Vitamin B6	.005 mg	Alcohol	0 g
Vitamin B12	0 mcg	Caffeine	0 mg
Folate	1.23 mcg	Water	7.62 g

☺ Avocado Pie

Calories	238	Pantothenic	.781 mg
Protein	4.91 g	Vitamin C	6.73 mg
Carbohydrates	27 g	Vitamin D	.045 mcg
Fat—Total	13.4 g	Vitamin E-Alpha E	1.24 mg
Saturated Fat	5.38 g	Calcium	115 mg
Monounsaturated Fat	5.92 g	Copper	.161 mg
Polyunsaturated Fat	1.17 g	Iron	.613 mg
Omega 3 Fatty Acid	.124 g	Magnesium	30 mg
Omega 6 Fatty Acid	1.04 g	Manganese	.123 mg
Cholesterol	13 mg	Phosphorus	119 mg
Dietary Fiber	2.08 g	Potassium	450 mg
Total Vitamin A	69.9 RE	Selenium	.656 mcg
A–Retinol	27.9 RE	Sodium	57.8 mg
A–Carotenoi	42 RE	Zinc	.577 mg
Thiamin–B1	.09 mg	Complex Carbohydrates	1.21 g
Riboflavin–B2	.222 mg	Sugars	23.7 g
Niacin–B3	1.05 mg	Mono-Saccharide	.433 g
Niacin Equivalent	1.05 mg	Di-Saccharide	20.8 g
Vitamin B6	.162 mg	Alcohol	0 g
Vitamin B12	.17 mcg	Caffeine	0 mg
Folate	36.1 mcg	Water	56.1 g

☺ Banana Cookies

Calories	29.2	Pantothenic	.029 mg
Protein	.698 g	Vitamin C	.096 mg
Carbohydrates	4.82 g	Vitamin D	.24 mcg
Fat—Total	.851 g	Vitamin E-Alpha E	.121 mg
Saturated Fat	.131 g	Calcium	1.27 mg
Monounsaturated Fat	.259 g	Copper	.012 mg
Polyunsaturated Fat	.283 g	Iron	.308 mg
Omega 3 Fatty Acid	.005 g	Magnesium	2.77 mg
Omega 6 Fatty Acid	.279 g	Manganese	.028 mg
Cholesterol	2.96 mg	Phosphorus	10.9 mg
Dietary Fiber	.275 g	Potassium	15.5 mg
Total Vitamin A	26.5 RE	Selenium	1.94 mcg
A–Retinol	15.7 RE	Sodium	10.3 mg
A–Carotenoi	1.37 RE	Zinc	.273 mg
Thiamin–B1	.055 mg	Complex Carbohydrates	3.7 g
Riboflavin–B2	.051 mg	Sugars	.842 g
Niacin–B3	.552 mg	Mono-Saccharide	.123 g
Niacin Equivalent	.237 mg	Di-Saccharide	.124 g
Vitamin B6	.04 mg	Alcohol	0 g
Vitamin B12	.103 mcg	Caffeine	0 mg
Folate	7.87 mcg	Water	2.74 g

⊚ Blueberry Cake

Calories	68.6	Pantothenic	.134 mg
Protein	1.47 g	Vitamin C	4.51 mg
Carbohydrates	7.96 g	Vitamin D	.438 mcg
Fat—Total	3.52 g	Vitamin E-Alpha E	.354 mg
Saturated Fat	1.78 g	Calcium	5.74 mg
Monounsaturated Fat	.775 g	Copper	.037 mg
Polyunsaturated Fat	.701 g	Iron	.722 mg
Omega 3 Fatty Acid	.013 g	Magnesium	5 mg
Omega 6 Fatty Acid	.679 g	Manganese	.13 mg
Cholesterol	20 mg	Phosphorus	22 mg
Dietary Fiber	.684 g	Potassium	47.2 mg
Total Vitamin A	46.2 RE	Selenium	2.22 mcg
A–Retinol	41.2 RE	Sodium	19.8 mg
A–Carotenoi	4.9 RE	Zinc	.157 mg
Thiamin–B1	.081 mg	Complex Carbohydrates	5.59 g
Riboflavin–B2	.064 mg	Sugars	1.7 g
Niacin–B3	.575 mg	Mono-Saccharide	.83 g
Niacin Equivalent	.575 mg	Di-Saccharide	.328 g
Vitamin B6	.021 mg	Alcohol	0 g
Vitamin B12	.049 mcg	Caffeine	0 mg
Folate	6.51 mcg	Water	17.3 g

⊚ Bon Bons

Calories	31.4	Pantothenic	.017 mg
Protein	.968 g	Vitamin C	.026 mg
Carbohydrates	3.86 g	Vitamin D	.002 mcg
Fat—Total	1.39 g	Vitamin E-Alpha E	.004 mg
Saturated Fat	1.18 g	Calcium	40.5 mg
Monounsaturated Fat	.041 g	Copper	0 mg
Polyunsaturated Fat	.005 g	Iron	.055 mg
Omega 3 Fatty Acid	.002 g	Magnesium	.495 mg
Omega 6 Fatty Acid	.003 g	Manganese	0 mg
Cholesterol	.916 mg	Phosphorus	3.6 mg
Dietary Fiber	.003 g	Potassium	6.95 mg
Total Vitamin A	1.91 RE	Selenium	.126 mcg
A–Retinol	1.4 RE	Sodium	2.81 mg
A–Carotenoi	.155 RE	Zinc	.015 mg
Thiamin–B1	.002 mg	Complex Carbohydrates	.003 g
Riboflavin–B2	.009 mg	Sugars	2.7 g
Niacin–B3	.003 mg	Mono-Saccharide	0 g
Niacin Equivalent	.003 mg	Di-Saccharide	0 g
Vitamin B6	.002 mg	Alcohol	0 g
Vitamin B12	.022 mcg	Caffeine	0 mg
Folate	.198 mcg	Water	2.25 g

⑨ Bread Pudding

Calories	161	Pantothenic	1.27 mg
Protein	9.59 g	Vitamin C	.811 mg
Carbohydrates	22.5 g	Vitamin D	1.61 mcg
Fat—Total	3.38 g	Vitamin E-Alpha E	.535 mg
Saturated Fat	.696 g	Calcium	173 mg
Monounsaturated Fat	1.16 g	Copper	.091 mg
Polyunsaturated Fat	1.28 g	Iron	1.52 mg
Omega 3 Fatty Acid	.075 g	Magnesium	23.5 mg
Omega 6 Fatty Acid	1.2 g	Manganese	.16 mg
Cholesterol	1.99 mg	Phosphorus	162 mg
Dietary Fiber	2.44 g	Potassium	324 mg
Total Vitamin A	159 RE	Selenium	10.2 mcg
A–Retinol	88.1 RE	Sodium	279 mg
A–Carotenoi	70.7 RE	Zinc	1.07 mg
Thiamin–B1	.203 mg	Complex Carbohydrates	12.6 g
Riboflavin–B2	.336 mg	Sugars	5.32 g
Niacin–B3	1.44 mg	Mono-Saccharide	0 g
Niacin Equivalent	1.45 mg	Di-Saccharide	4.79 g
Vitamin B6	.061 mg	Alcohol	0 g
Vitamin B12	.365 mcg	Caffeine	0 mg
Folate	18.7 mcg	Water	105 g

⑨ Brownies

Calories	38.2	Pantothenic	.02 mg
Protein	.852 g	Vitamin C	.016 mg
Carbohydrates	4.03 g	Vitamin D	.001 mcg
Fat—Total	2.09 g	Vitamin E-Alpha E	.919 mg
Saturated Fat	.655 g	Calcium	23.4 mg
Monounsaturated Fat	.325 g	Copper	.011 mg
Polyunsaturated Fat	1.01 g	Iron	.146 mg
Omega 3 Fatty Acid	.006 g	Magnesium	1.63 mg
Omega 6 Fatty Acid	1 g	Manganese	.019 mg
Cholesterol	.292 mg	Phosphorus	5.66 mg
Dietary Fiber	.626 g	Potassium	19.9 mg
Total Vitamin A	.439 RE	Selenium	1.03 mcg
A–Retinol	.238 RE	Sodium	4.32 mg
A–Carotenoi	.048 RE	Zinc	.041 mg
Thiamin–B1	.015 mg	Complex Carbohydrates	1.24 g
Riboflavin–B2	.026 mg	Sugars	.979 g
Niacin–B3	.133 mg	Mono-Saccharide	.061 g
Niacin Equivalent	.133 mg	Di-Saccharide	.085 g
Vitamin B6	.007 mg	Alcohol	0 g
Vitamin B12	.013 mcg	Caffeine	0 mg
Folate	1.1 mcg	Water	3.09 g

⑨ Buckeyes

Calories	61.2	Pantothenic	.056 mg
Protein	2.1 g	Vitamin C	.001 mg
Carbohydrates	2.63 g	Vitamin D	0 mcg
Fat—Total	5.06 g	Vitamin E-Alpha E	.194 mg
Saturated Fat	1.39 g	Calcium	21.5 mg
Monounsaturated Fat	1.98 g	Copper	.039 mg
Polyunsaturated Fat	1.25 g	Iron	.142 mg
Omega 3 Fatty Acid	.009 g	Magnesium	10.9 mg
Omega 6 Fatty Acid	1.24 g	Manganese	.097 mg
Cholesterol	.242 mg	Phosphorus	21.4 mg
Dietary Fiber	.399 g	Potassium	42.3 mg
Total Vitamin A	15.2 RE	Selenium	0 mcg
A–Retinol	13.8 RE	Sodium	1.06 mg
A–Carotenoi	1.24 RE	Zinc	.181 mg
Thiamin–B1	.01 mg	Complex Carbohydrates	.376 g
Riboflavin–B2	.006 mg	Sugars	1.52 g
Niacin–B3	.858 mg	Mono-Saccharide	.073 g
Niacin Equivalent	.858 mg	Di-Saccharide	.399 g
Vitamin B6	.027 mg	Alcohol	0 g
Vitamin B12	.001 mcg	Caffeine	0 mg
Folate	4.74 mcg	Water	.353 g

⑨ Butter Crunch

Calories	28.4	Pantothenic	.021 mg
Protein	.339 g	Vitamin C	.003 mg
Carbohydrates	.348 g	Vitamin D	0 mcg
Fat—Total	2.96 g	Vitamin E-Alpha E	.465 mg
Saturated Fat	.521 g	Calcium	1.23 mg
Monounsaturated Fat	1.38 g	Copper	.009 mg
Polyunsaturated Fat	.925 g	Iron	.031 mg
Omega 3 Fatty Acid	.009 g	Magnesium	2.44 mg
Omega 6 Fatty Acid	.917 g	Manganese	.029 mg
Cholesterol	0 mg	Phosphorus	5.32 mg
Dietary Fiber	.095 g	Potassium	9.71 mg
Total Vitamin A	28.2 RE	Selenium	.101 mcg
A–Retinol	25.8 RE	Sodium	.322 mg
A–Carotenoi	2.32 RE	Zinc	.045 mg
Thiamin–B1	.006 mg	Complex Carbohydrates	.137 g
Riboflavin–B2	.002 mg	Sugars	.077 g
Niacin–B3	.185 mg	Mono-Saccharide	.003 g
Niacin Equivalent	.185 mg	Di-Saccharide	.055 g
Vitamin B6	.004 mg	Alcohol	0 g
Vitamin B12	.002 mcg	Caffeine	0 mg
Folate	2.01 mcg	Water	.595 g

⊚ Candied Nuts

Calories	40.9	Pantothenic	.03 mg
Protcin	.636 g	Vitamin C	.143 mg
Carbohydrates	4.17 g	Vitamin D	0 mcg
Fat—Total	2.75 g	Vitamin E-Alpha E	.116 mg
Saturated Fat	.248 g	Calcium	4.25 mg
Monounsaturated Fat	.631 g	Copper	.062 mg
Polyunsaturated Fat	1.74 g	Iron	.11 mg
Omega 3 Fatty Acid	.303 g	Magnesium	7.51 mg
Omega 6 Fatty Acid	1.41 g	Manganese	.136 mg
Cholesterol	0 mg	Phosphorus	17.3 mg
Dietary Fiber	.201 g	Potassium	22.5 mg
Total Vitamin A	.551 RE	Selenium	.222 mcg
A–Retinol	0 RE	Sodium	15.6 mg
A–Carotenoi	.551 RE	Zinc	.123 mg
Thiamin–B1	.018 mg	Complex Carbohydrates	.52 g
Riboflavin–B2	.007 mg	Sugars	.097 g
Niacin–B3	.048 mg	Mono-Saccharide	0 g
Niacin Equivalent	.048 mg	Di-Saccharide	.093 g
Vitamin B6	.025 mg	Alcohol	0 g
Vitamin B12	0 mcg	Caffeine	0 mg
Folate	2.93 mcg	Water	4.31 g

⊚ Candied Prunes

Calories	13.7	Pantothenic	.026 mg
Protein	.148 g	Vitamin C	.187 mg
Carbohydrates	3.6 g	Vitamin D	0 mcg
Fat—Total	.029 g	Vitamin E-Alpha E	.076 mg
Saturated Fat	.002 g	Calcium	2.93 mg
Monounsaturated Fat	.019 g	Copper	.025 mg
Polyunsaturated Fat	.006 g	Iron	.146 mg
Omega 3 Fatty Acid	0 g	Magnesium	2.72 mg
Omega 6 Fatty Acid	.006 g	Manganese	.013 mg
Cholesterol	0 mg	Phosphorus	4.55 mg
Dietary Fiber	.524 g	Potassium	43 mg
Total Vitamin A	11.3 RE	Selenium	.152 mcg
A–Retinol	0 RE	Sodium	.234 mg
A–Carotenoi	11.3 RE	Zinc	.03 mg
Thiamin–B1	.005 mg	Complex Carbohydrates	0 g
Riboflavin–B2	.009 mg	Sugars	2.48 g
Niacin–B3	.111 mg	Mono-Saccharide	2.11 g
Niacin Equivalent	.111 mg	Di-Saccharide	.045 g
Vitamin B6	.015 mg	Alcohol	0 g
Vitamin B12	0 mcg	Caffeine	0 mg
Folate	.21 mcg	Water	2.54 g

☺ Carob Chip Cookies

Calories	59	Pantothenic	.035 mg
Protein	1.76 g	Vitamin C	.002 mg
Carbohydrates	7.33 g	Vitamin D	.186 mcg
Fat—Total	2.52 g	Vitamin E-Alpha E	.125 mg
Saturated Fat	1.67 g	Calcium	51.4 mg
Monounsaturated Fat	.285 g	Copper	.006 mg
Polyunsaturated Fat	.292 g	Iron	.273 mg
Omega 3 Fatty Acid	.005 g	Magnesium	1.02 mg
Omega 6 Fatty Acid	.288 g	Manganese	.027 mg
Cholesterol	6.55 mg	Phosphorus	6.91 mg
Dietary Fiber	.128 g	Potassium	6.27 mg
Total Vitamin A	18.8 RE	Selenium	1.75 mcg
A–Retinol	17 RE	Sodium	7.38 mg
A–Carotenoi	1.29 RE	Zinc	.043 mg
Thiamin–B1	.032 mg	Complex Carbohydrates	2.78 g
Riboflavin–B2	.027 mg	Sugars	2.8 g
Niacin–B3	.232 mg	Mono-Saccharide	.052 g
Niacin Equivalent	.232 mg	Di-Saccharide	.016 g
Vitamin B6	.004 mg	Alcohol	0 g
Vitamin B12	.015 mcg	Caffeine	0 mg
Folate	1.68 mcg	Water	2.43 g

☺ Carob and Coconut Macaroons

Calories	56.1	Pantothenic	.07 mg
Protein	1.28 g	Vitamin C	.074 mg
Carbohydrates	3.56 g	Vitamin D	.032 mcg
Fat—Total	4.33 g	Vitamin E-Alpha E	.091 mg
Saturated Fat	3.69 g	Calcium	29.4 mg
Monounsaturated Fat	.23 g	Copper	.039 mg
Polyunsaturated Fat	.068 g	Iron	.238 mg
Omega 3 Fatty Acid	.002 g	Magnesium	4.64 mg
Omega 6 Fatty Acid	.067 g	Manganese	.135 mg
Cholesterol	11 mg	Phosphorus	14.5 mg
Dietary Fiber	.838 g	Potassium	33 mg
Total Vitamin A	5.05 RE	Selenium	1.55 mcg
A–Retinol	4.78 RE	Sodium	4.97 mg
A–Carotenoi	0 RE	Zinc	.127 mg
Thiamin–B1	.004 mg	Complex Carbohydrates	.013 g
Riboflavin–B2	.018 mg	Sugars	1.88 g
Niacin–B3	.031 mg	Mono-Saccharide	.031 g
Niacin Equivalent	.031 mg	Di-Saccharide	0 g
Vitamin B6	.018 mg	Alcohol	0 g
Vitamin B12	.025 mcg	Caffeine	0 mg
Folate	1.61 mcg	Water	2.03 g

⊚ Carrott Cake

Calories	35.9	Pantothenic	.052 mg
Protein	.829 g	Vitamin C	1.26 mg
Carbohydrates	8.02 g	Vitamin D	.012 mcg
Fat—Total	.095 g	Vitamin E-Alpha E	.071 mg
Saturated Fat	.017 g	Calcium	7.04 mg
Monounsaturated Fat	.008 g	Copper	.028 mg
Polyunsaturated Fat	.036 g	Iron	.417 mg
Omega 3 Fatty Acid	.004 g	Magnesium	4.42 mg
Omega 6 Fatty Acid	.032 g	Manganese	.18 mg
Cholesterol	.022 mg	Phosphorus	12.6 mg
Dietary Fiber	.496 g	Potassium	46.3 mg
Total Vitamin A	125 RE	Selenium	2.44 mcg
A–Retinol	.745 RE	Sodium	52.9 mg
A–Carotenoi	124 RE	Zinc	.077 mg
Thiamin–B1	.063 mg	Complex Carbohydrates	4.51 g
Riboflavin–B2	.041 mg	Sugars	3.02 g
Niacin–B3	.46 mg	Mono-Saccharide	1.22 g
Niacin Equivalent	.459 mg	Di-Saccharide	.243 g
Vitamin B6	.023 mg	Alcohol	0 g
Vitamin B12	.005 mcg	Caffeine	0 mg
Folate	2.83 mcg	Water	14.7 g

⊚ Cherries à la Fudge

Calories	33.5	Pantothenic	0 mg
Protein	1.13 g	Vitamin C	0 mg
Carbohydrates	4.53 g	Vitamin D	0 mcg
Fat—Total	1.25 g	Vitamin E-Alpha E	.006 mg
Saturated Fat	1.1 g	Calcium	36.5 mg
Monounsaturated Fat	.002 g	Copper	.005 mg
Polyunsaturated Fat	.002 g	Iron	.064 mg
Omega 3 Fatty Acid	.001 g	Magnesium	.005 mg
Omega 6 Fatty Acid	.001 g	Manganese	0 mg
Cholesterol	.454 mg	Phosphorus	7 mg
Dietary Fiber	0 g	Potassium	5.43 mg
Total Vitamin A	.365 RE	Selenium	0 mcg
A–Retinol	0 RE	Sodium	10.9 mg
A–Carotenoi	0 RE	Zinc	0 mg
Thiamin–B1	0 mg	Complex Carbohydrates	0 g
Riboflavin–B2	.001 mg	Sugars	1.95 g
Niacin–B3	0 mg	Mono-Saccharide	0 g
Niacin Equivalent	0 mg	Di-Saccharide	0 g
Vitamin B6	0 mg	Alcohol	0 g
Vitamin B12	0 mcg	Caffeine	0 mg
Folate	.07 mcg	Water	3.01 g

☺ Cherry Cheesecake

Calories	66.3	Pantothenic	.326 mg
Protein	4.37 g	Vitamin C	4.21 mg
Carbohydrates	12 g	Vitamin D	.737 mcg
Fat—Total	.129 g	Vitamin E-Alpha E	.035 mg
Saturated Fat	.058 g	Calcium	112 mg
Monounsaturated Fat	.036 g	Copper	.041 mg
Polyunsaturated Fat	.022 g	Iron	.75 mg
Omega 3 Fatty Acid	.009 g	Magnesium	13.1 mg
Omega 6 Fatty Acid	.013 g	Manganese	.039 mg
Cholesterol	2.82 mg	Phosphorus	77.1 mg
Dietary Fiber	.416 g	Potassium	175 mg
Total Vitamin A	101 RE	Selenium	1.23 mcg
A–Retinol	43.1 RE	Sodium	96.8 mg
A–Carotenoi	34.3 RE	Zinc	.369 mg
Thiamin–B1	.026 mg	Complex Carbohydrates	2.89 g
Riboflavin–B2	.15 mg	Sugars	8.41 g
Niacin–B3	.151 mg	Mono-Saccharide	.128 g
Niacin Equivalent	.145 mg	Di-Saccharide	4.22 g
Vitamin B6	.043 mg	Alcohol	0 g
Vitamin B12	.088 mcg	Caffeine	0 mg
Folate	7.58 mcg	Water	75.9 g

☺ Cherry Fudge

Calories	34.6	Pantothenic	.016 mg
Protein	.231 g	Vitamin C	.399 mg
Carbohydrates	.651 g	Vitamin D	.011 mcg
Fat—Total	3.56 g	Vitamin E-Alpha E	.465 mg
Saturated Fat	.747 g	Calcium	4.52 mg
Monounsaturated Fat	1.45 g	Copper	.013 mg
Polyunsaturated Fat	1.2 g	Iron	.028 mg
Omega 3 Fatty Acid	.075 g	Magnesium	1.9 mg
Omega 6 Fatty Acid	1.12 g	Manganese	.026 mg
Cholesterol	.992 mg	Phosphorus	6.04 mg
Dietary Fiber	.043 g	Potassium	13.5 mg
Total Vitamin A	36.5 RE	Selenium	.094 mcg
A–Retinol	33.1 RE	Sodium	1.28 mg
A–Carotenoi	3.31 RE	Zinc	.038 mg
Thiamin–B1	.005 mg	Complex Carbohydrates	.122 g
Riboflavin–B2	.006 mg	Sugars	.208 g
Niacin–B3	.014 mg	Mono-Saccharide	.031 g
Niacin Equivalent	.014 mg	Di-Saccharide	.156 g
Vitamin B6	.007 mg	Alcohol	0 g
Vitamin B12	.011 mcg	Caffeine	0 mg
Folate	.854 mcg	Water	4.02 g

☺ Cherry Coconut Macaroons

Calories	34.1	Pantothenic	.042 mg
Protein	.546 g	Vitamin C	.076 mg
Carbohydrates	1.26 g	Vitamin D	0 mcg
Fat—Total	3.23 g	Vitamin E-Alpha E	.07 mg
Saturated Fat	2.87 g	Calcium	1.42 mg
Monounsaturated Fat	.138 g	Copper	.04 mg
Polyunsaturated Fat	.035 g	Iron	.169 mg
Omega 3 Fatty Acid	0 g	Magnesium	4.72 mg
Omega 6 Fatty Acid	.035 g	Manganese	.138 mg
Cholesterol	0 mg	Phosphorus	10.6 mg
Dietary Fiber	.862 g	Potassium	33.9 mg
Total Vitamin A	0 RE	Selenium	1.14 mcg
A–Retinol	0 RE	Sodium	5 mg
A–Carotenoi	0 RE	Zinc	.102 mg
Thiamin–B1	.003 mg	Complex Carbohydrates	.014 g
Riboflavin–B2	.014 mg	Sugars	.416 g
Niacin–B3	.032 mg	Mono-Saccharide	.02 g
Niacin Equivalent	.032 mg	Di-Saccharide	0 g
Vitamin B6	.015 mg	Alcohol	0 g
Vitamin B12	.004 mcg	Caffeine	0 mg
Folate	.509 mcg	Water	1.83 g

☺ Cherry Scones

Calories	110	Pantothenic	.165 mg
Protein	2.75 g	Vitamin C	.273 mg
Carbohydrates	21.1 g	Vitamin D	.27 mcg
Fat—Total	2.73 g	Vitamin E-Alpha E	1.19 mg
Saturated Fat	.4 g	Calcium	46.8 mg
Monounsaturated Fat	.665 g	Copper	.072 mg
Polyunsaturated Fat	1.5 g	Iron	.881 mg
Omega 3 Fatty Acid	.015 g	Magnesium	12.5 mg
Omega 6 Fatty Acid	1.49 g	Manganese	.145 mg
Cholesterol	.56 mg	Phosphorus	72.1 mg
Dietary Fiber	1.05 g	Potassium	105 mg
Total Vitamin A	68.6 RE	Selenium	5.68 mcg
A–Retinol	21.5 RE	Sodium	21.8 mg
A–Carotenoi	2.45 RE	Zinc	.245 mg
Thiamin–B1	.129 mg	Complex Carbohydrates	11.3 g
Riboflavin–B2	.119 mg	Sugars	1.1 g
Niacin–B3	.949 mg	Mono-Saccharide	.248 g
Niacin Equivalent	.893 mg	Di-Saccharide	.743 g
Vitamin B6	.017 mg	Alcohol	0 g
Vitamin B12	.046 mcg	Caffeine	0 mg
Folate	5.07 mcg	Water	15.6 g

ᴑ Chocolate Bars

Calories	54.2	Pantothenic	.026 mg
Protein	1.35 g	Vitamin C	.003 mg
Carbohydrates	6.12 g	Vitamin D	.344 mcg
Fat—Total	2.72 g	Vitamin E-Alpha E	.215 mg
Saturated Fat	1.45 g	Calcium	41.3 mg
Monounsaturated Fat	.488 g	Copper	.005 mg
Polyunsaturated Fat	.537 g	Iron	.227 mg
Omega 3 Fatty Acid	.008 g	Magnesium	.834 mg
Omega 6 Fatty Acid	.532 g	Manganese	.024 mg
Cholesterol	3.46 mg	Phosphorus	5.31 mg
Dietary Fiber	.114 g	Potassium	4.74 mg
Total Vitamin A	33.1 RE	Selenium	1.28 mcg
A–Retinol	30 RE	Sodium	11.3 mg
A–Carotenoi	2.58 RE	Zinc	.031 mg
Thiamin–B1	.028 mg	Complex Carbohydrates	2.48 g
Riboflavin–B2	.019 mg	Sugars	2.24 g
Niacin–B3	.205 mg	Mono-Saccharide	.036 g
Niacin Equivalent	.205 mg	Di-Saccharide	.014 g
Vitamin B6	.003 mg	Alcohol	0 g
Vitamin B12	.009 mcg	Caffeine	0 mg
Folate	1.26 mcg	Water	2.36 g

ᴑ Chocolate Cake

Calories	54.3	Pantothenic	.094 mg
Protein	1.47 g	Vitamin C	.102 mg
Carbohydrates	7.95 g	Vitamin D	.159 mcg
Fat—Total	1.8 g	Vitamin E-Alpha E	1.05 mg
Saturated Fat	.222 g	Calcium	28.5 mg
Monounsaturated Fat	.367 g	Copper	.019 mg
Polyunsaturated Fat	1.16 g	Iron	.422 mg
Omega 3 Fatty Acid	.008 g	Magnesium	4.52 mg
Omega 6 Fatty Acid	1.15 g	Manganese	.06 mg
Cholesterol	.287 mg	Phosphorus	24.9 mg
Dietary Fiber	.736 g	Potassium	44.8 mg
Total Vitamin A	9.32 RE	Selenium	2.93 mcg
A–Retinol	9.31 RE	Sodium	9.74 mg
A–Carotenoi	.012 RE	Zinc	.138 mg
Thiamin–B1	.066 mg	Complex Carbohydrates	5.57 g
Riboflavin–B2	.069 mg	Sugars	1.04 g
Niacin–B3	.498 mg	Mono-Saccharide	.071 g
Niacin Equivalent	.498 mg	Di-Saccharide	.941 g
Vitamin B6	.012 mg	Alcohol	0 g
Vitamin B12	.019 mcg	Caffeine	0 mg
Folate	3.07 mcg	Water	7.3 g

☺ Chocolate Peanut Butter Fudge

Calories	33.5	Pantothenic	.021 mg
Protein	1.12 g	Vitamin C	.111 mg
Carbohydrates	3.37 g	Vitamin D	0 mcg
Fat—Total	1.82 g	Vitamin E-Alpha E	.107 mg
Saturated Fat	1.11 g	Calcium	32.6 mg
Monounsaturated Fat	.336 g	Copper	.01 mg
Polyunsaturated Fat	.206 g	Iron	.077 mg
Omega 3 Fatty Acid	.001 g	Magnesium	2.56 mg
Omega 6 Fatty Acid	.204 g	Manganese	.029 mg
Cholesterol	.403 mg	Phosphorus	5.09 mg
Dietary Fiber	.114 g	Potassium	15.5 mg
Total Vitamin A	.324 RE	Selenium	.119 mcg
A–Retinol	0 RE	Sodium	.317 mg
A–Carotenoi	0 RE	Zinc	.044 mg
Thiamin–B1	.003 mg	Complex Carbohydrates	.356 g
Riboflavin–B2	.002 mg	Sugars	1.86 g
Niacin–B3	.214 mg	Mono-Saccharide	.017 g
Niacin Equivalent	.214 mg	Di-Saccharide	.094 g
Vitamin B6	.01 mg	Alcohol	0 g
Vitamin B12	0 mcg	Caffeine	0 mg
Folate	1.44 mcg	Water	1.18 g

☺ Chocolate Soufflé

Calories	40.2	Pantothenic	.044 mg
Protein	.333 g	Vitamin C	.312 mg
Carbohydrates	10.3 g	Vitamin D	0 mcg
Fat—Total	.059 g	Vitamin E-Alpha E	.126 mg
Saturated Fat	.005 g	Calcium	6.33 mg
Monounsaturated Fat	.035 g	Copper	.043 mg
Polyunsaturated Fat	.014 g	Iron	.453 mg
Omega 3 Fatty Acid	0 g	Magnesium	4.49 mg
Omega 6 Fatty Acid	.014 g	Manganese	.024 mg
Cholesterol	0 mg	Phosphorus	7.8 mg
Dietary Fiber	1.54 g	Potassium	75.3 mg
Total Vitamin A	18.8 RE	Selenium	.247 mcg
A–Retinol	0 RE	Sodium	5.26 mg
A–Carotenoi	18.8 RE	Zinc	.054 mg
Thiamin–B1	.008 mg	Complex Carbohydrates	0 g
Riboflavin–B2	.015 mg	Sugars	4.06 g
Niacin–B3	.221 mg	Mono-Saccharide	3.51 g
Niacin Equivalent	.186 mg	Di-Saccharide	.076 g
Vitamin B6	.031 mg	Alcohol	0 g
Vitamin B12	0 mcg	Caffeine	0 mg
Folate	.35 mcg	Water	3.2 g

✪ Christmas Trees

Calories	58.1	Pantothenic	.011 mg
Protein	1.38 g	Vitamin C	.105 mg
Carbohydrates	5.15 g	Vitamin D	.001 mcg
Fat—Total	3.68 g	Vitamin E-Alpha E	.119 mg
Saturated Fat	2.79 g	Calcium	54.9 mg
Monounsaturated Fat	.371 g	Copper	.013 mg
Polyunsaturated Fat	.195 g	Iron	.15 mg
Omega 3 Fatty Acid	.004 g	Magnesium	1.02 mg
Omega 6 Fatty Acid	.191 g	Manganese	.045 mg
Cholesterol	1.51 mg	Phosphorus	3.94 mg
Dietary Fiber	.282 g	Potassium	11.6 mg
Total Vitamin A	9.8 RE	Selenium	.597 mcg
A–Retinol	8.5 RE	Sodium	.872 mg
A–Carotenoi	.737 RE	Zinc	.035 mg
Thiamin–B1	.002 mg	Complex Carbohydrates	0 g
Riboflavin–B2	.002 mg	Sugars	3.14 g
Niacin–B3	.017 mg	Mono-Saccharide	.102 g
Niacin Equivalent	.017 mg	Di-Saccharide	.025 g
Vitamin B6	.002 mg	Alcohol	0 g
Vitamin B12	.002 mcg	Caffeine	0 mg
Folate	.824 mcg	Water	2.02 g

✪ Cinnamon Bon Bons

Calories	37.9	Pantothenic	.073 mg
Protein	1.04 g	Vitamin C	.817 mg
Carbohydrates	4.44 g	Vitamin D	.032 mcg
Fat—Total	1.86 g	Vitamin E-Alpha E	.067 mg
Saturated Fat	.8 g	Calcium	29.3 mg
Monounsaturated Fat	.279 g	Copper	.038 mg
Polyunsaturated Fat	.635 g	Iron	.106 mg
Omega 3 Fatty Acid	.104 g	Magnesium	5 mg
Omega 6 Fatty Acid	.525 g	Manganese	.058 mg
Cholesterol	.341 mg	Phosphorus	12 mg
Dietary Fiber	.2 g	Potassium	52.7 mg
Total Vitamin A	4.04 RE	Selenium	.193 mcg
A–Retinol	3.48 RE	Sodium	2.5 mg
A–Carotenoi	.331 RE	Zinc	.083 mg
Thiamin–B1	.016 mg	Complex Carbohydrates	1.93 g
Riboflavin–B2	.009 mg	Sugars	1.54 g
Niacin–B3	.151 mg	Mono-Saccharide	0 g
Niacin Equivalent	.151 mg	Di-Saccharide	.213 g
Vitamin B6	.036 mg	Alcohol	0 g
Vitamin B12	.004 mcg	Caffeine	0 mg
Folate	2.03 mcg	Water	9.26 g

☺ Citrus Candy

Calories	3.33	Pantothenic	.019 mg
Protein	.061 g	Vitamin C	5.44 mg
Carbohydrates	1 g	Vitamin D	0 mcg
Fat—Total	.008 g	Vitamin E-Alpha E	.016 mg
Saturated Fat	.001 g	Calcium	6.44 mg
Monounsaturated Fat	.001 g	Copper	.003 mg
Polyunsaturated Fat	.001 g	Iron	.032 mg
Omega 3 Fatty Acid	.001 g	Magnesium	.88 mg
Omega 6 Fatty Acid	.001 g	Manganese	0 mg
Cholesterol	0 mg	Phosphorus	.84 mg
Dietary Fiber	.136 g	Potassium	8.47 mg
Total Vitamin A	1.68 RE	Selenium	.003 mcg
A–Retinol	0 RE	Sodium	.12 mg
A–Carotenoi	1.68 RE	Zinc	.01 mg
Thiamin–B1	.005 mg	Complex Carbohydrates	.867 g
Riboflavin–B2	.003 mg	Sugars	0 g
Niacin–B3	.036 mg	Mono-Saccharide	0 g
Niacin Equivalent	0 mg	Di-Saccharide	0 g
Vitamin B6	.007 mg	Alcohol	0 g
Vitamin B12	0 mcg	Caffeine	0 mg
Folate	1.2 mcg	Water	2.9 g

☺ Coated Citrus Candy

Calories	19.2	Pantothenic	.008 mg
Protein	.586 g	Vitamin C	2.18 mg
Carbohydrates	2.47 g	Vitamin D	0 mcg
Fat—Total	.835 g	Vitamin E-Alpha E	.006 mg
Saturated Fat	.731 g	Calcium	26.5 mg
Monounsaturated Fat	.001 g	Copper	.001 mg
Polyunsaturated Fat	.001 g	Iron	.047 mg
Omega 3 Fatty Acid	0 g	Magnesium	.352 mg
Omega 6 Fatty Acid	.001 g	Manganese	0 mg
Cholesterol	.302 mg	Phosphorus	.336 mg
Dietary Fiber	.054 g	Potassium	3.39 mg
Total Vitamin A	.915 RE	Selenium	.001 mcg
A–Retinol	0 RE	Sodium	.048 mg
A–Carotenoi	.672 RE	Zinc	.004 mg
Thiamin–B1	.002 mg	Complex Carbohydrates	.347 g
Riboflavin–B2	.001 mg	Sugars	1.3 g
Niacin–B3	.014 mg	Mono-Saccharide	0 g
Niacin Equivalent	0 mg	Di-Saccharide	0 g
Vitamin B6	.003 mg	Alcohol	0 g
Vitamin B12	0 mcg	Caffeine	0 mg
Folate	.48 mcg	Water	1.16 g

◎ Cocoa Balls

Calories	19.5	Pantothenic	.045 mg
Protein	.453 g	Vitamin C	.085 mg
Carbohydrates	1.87 g	Vitamin D	.002 mcg
Fat—Total	1.37 g	Vitamin E-Alpha E	.053 mg
Saturated Fat	.268 g	Calcium	7.47 mg
Monounsaturated Fat	.759 g	Copper	.052 mg
Polyunsaturated Fat	.276 g	Iron	.158 mg
Omega 3 Fatty Acid	.013 g	Magnesium	6.84 mg
Omega 6 Fatty Acid	.262 g	Manganese	.105 mg
Cholesterol	.693 mg	Phosphorus	16.1 mg
Dietary Fiber	.36 g	Potassium	26.9 mg
Total Vitamin A	1.87 RE	Selenium	.28 mcg
A–Retinol	1.49 RE	Sodium	2.79 mg
A–Carotenoi	.383 RE	Zinc	.165 mg
Thiamin–B1	.016 mg	Complex Carbohydrates	.312 g
Riboflavin–B2	.013 mg	Sugars	1.2 g
Niacin–B3	.037 mg	Mono-Saccharide	.005 g
Niacin Equivalent	.037 mg	Di-Saccharide	1.17 g
Vitamin B6	.005 mg	Alcohol	0 g
Vitamin B12	.009 mcg	Caffeine	1.98 mg
Folate	1.13 mcg	Water	.761 g

◎ Coconut Crisps

Calories	8.4	Pantothenic	.012 mg
Protein	.134 g	Vitamin C	.085 mg
Carbohydrates	.401 g	Vitamin D	.02 mcg
Fat—Total	.738 g	Vitamin E-Alpha E	.016 mg
Saturated Fat	.637 g	Calcium	2.7 mg
Monounsaturated Fat	.048 g	Copper	.009 mg
Polyunsaturated Fat	.01 g	Iron	.05 mg
Omega 3 Fatty Acid	.001 g	Magnesium	.913 mg
Omega 6 Fatty Acid	.009 g	Manganese	.03 mg
Cholesterol	.277 mg	Phosphorus	4.16 mg
Dietary Fiber	.188 g	Potassium	10.2 mg
Total Vitamin A	.63 RE	Selenium	.436 mcg
A–Retinol	.549 RE	Sodium	1.4 mg
A–Carotenoi	.061 RE	Zinc	.03 mg
Thiamin–B1	.002 mg	Complex Carbohydrates	0 g
Riboflavin–B2	.004 mg	Sugars	.22 g
Niacin–B3	.013 mg	Mono-Saccharide	.068 g
Niacin Equivalent	.013 mg	Di-Saccharide	.097 g
Vitamin B6	.002 mg	Alcohol	0 g
Vitamin B12	.007 mcg	Caffeine	0 mg
Folate	.629 mcg	Water	2.75 g

◎ Coconut Delight

Calories	22.4	Pantothenic	.01 mg
Protein	.523 g	Vitamin C	.106 mg
Carbohydrates	1.74 g	Vitamin D	0 mcg
Fat—Total	1.57 g	Vitamin E-Alpha E	.023 mg
Saturated Fat	1.39 g	Calcium	14.8 mg
Monounsaturated Fat	.046 g	Copper	.014 mg
Polyunsaturated Fat	.012 g	Iron	.099 mg
Omega 3 Fatty Acid	0 g	Magnesium	1.11 mg
Omega 6 Fatty Acid	.012 g	Manganese	.048 mg
Cholesterol	.181 mg	Phosphorus	3.71 mg
Dietary Fiber	.301 g	Potassium	12.5 mg
Total Vitamin A	.146 RE	Selenium	.765 mcg
A–Retinol	0 RE	Sodium	1.88 mg
A–Carotenoi	0 RE	Zinc	.036 mg
Thiamin–B1	.002 mg	Complex Carbohydrates	0 g
Riboflavin–B2	.004 mg	Sugars	.986 g
Niacin–B3	.018 mg	Mono-Saccharide	.117 g
Niacin Equivalent	.018 mg	Di-Saccharide	.003 g
Vitamin B6	.002 mg	Alcohol	0 g
Vitamin B12	.002 mcg	Caffeine	0 mg
Folate	.867 mcg	Water	2.17 g

◎ Coconut Drops

Calories	19.2	Pantothenic	.016 mg
Protein	.291 g	Vitamin C	.096 mg
Carbohydrates	.509 g	Vitamin D	.005 mcg
Fat—Total	1.87 g	Vitamin E-Alpha E	.045 mg
Saturated Fat	1.42 g	Calcium	2.46 mg
Monounsaturated Fat	.295 g	Copper	.013 mg
Polyunsaturated Fat	.043 g	Iron	.101 mg
Omega 3 Fatty Acid	.013 g	Magnesium	1.09 mg
Omega 6 Fatty Acid	.031 g	Manganese	.043 mg
Cholesterol	2.83 mg	Phosphorus	5.94 mg
Dietary Fiber	.271 g	Potassium	13.4 mg
Total Vitamin A	11.3 RE	Selenium	.633 mcg
A–Retinol	10.7 RE	Sodium	8.21 mg
A–Carotenoi	.593 RE	Zinc	.046 mg
Thiamin–B1	.002 mg	Complex Carbohydrates	0 g
Riboflavin–B2	.006 mg	Sugars	.248 g
Niacin–B3	.018 mg	Mono-Saccharide	.098 g
Niacin Equivalent	.018 mg	Di-Saccharide	.047 g
Vitamin B6	.003 mg	Alcohol	0 g
Vitamin B12	.011 mcg	Caffeine	0 mg
Folate	1.1 mcg	Water	2.74 g

⑨ Coconut Rolls

Calories	10.9	Pantothenic	.004 mg
Protein	.038 g	Vitamin C	.018 mg
Carbohydrates	.086 g	Vitamin D	.002 mcg
Fat—Total	1.18 g	Vitamin E-Alpha E	.132 mg
Saturated Fat	.433 g	Calcium	.903 mg
Monounsaturated Fat	.443 g	Copper	.002 mg
Polyunsaturated Fat	.247 g	Iron	.008 mg
Omega 3 Fatty Acid	.006 g	Magnesium	.193 mg
Omega 6 Fatty Acid	.241 g	Manganese	.005 mg
Cholesterol	1.1 mg	Phosphorus	1.11 mg
Dietary Fiber	.031 g	Potassium	2.38 mg
Total Vitamin A	12.3 RE	Selenium	.072 mcg
A–Retinol	11.3 RE	Sodium	.43 mg
A–Carotenoi	.983 RE	Zinc	.006 mg
Thiamin–B1	.001 mg	Complex Carbohydrates	0 g
Riboflavin–B2	.002 mg	Sugars	.056 g
Niacin–B3	.002 mg	Mono-Saccharide	.011 g
Niacin Equivalent	.002 mg	Di-Saccharide	.03 g
Vitamin B6	.001 mg	Alcohol	0 g
Vitamin B12	.002 mcg	Caffeine	0 mg
Folate	.131 mcg	Water	.986 g

⑨ Coconut Sticks

Calories	51.6	Pantothenic	.068 mg
Protein	1.03 g	Vitamin C	.144 mg
Carbohydrates	8.21 g	Vitamin D	0 mcg
Fat—Total	2.17 g	Vitamin E-Alpha E	.817 mg
Saturated Fat	.486 g	Calcium	25.1 mg
Monounsaturated Fat	1.15 g	Copper	.07 mg
Polyunsaturated Fat	.425 g	Iron	.398 mg
Omega 3 Fatty Acid	.012 g	Magnesium	16.6 mg
Omega 6 Fatty Acid	.41 g	Manganese	.133 mg
Cholesterol	0 mg	Phosphorus	25.7 mg
Dietary Fiber	1.46 g	Potassium	108 mg
Total Vitamin A	1.51 RE	Selenium	1.03 mcg
A–Retinol	0 RE	Sodium	1.81 mg
A–Carotenoi	1.51 RE	Zinc	.164 mg
Thiamin–B1	.016 mg	Complex Carbohydrates	.172 g
Riboflavin–B2	.035 mg	Sugars	6.61 g
Niacin–B3	.193 mg	Mono-Saccharide	6.7 g
Niacin Equivalent	.194 mg	Di-Saccharide	.91 g
Vitamin B6	.03 mg	Alcohol	0 g
Vitamin B12	0 mcg	Caffeine	0 mg
Folate	3.02 mcg	Water	3.83 g

☉ Cranberry Banana Loaf Cake

Calories	64.4	Pantothenic	.084 mg
Protein	1.28 g	Vitamin C	1.61 mg
Carbohydrates	9.73 g	Vitamin D	0 mcg
Fat—Total	2.43 g	Vitamin E-Alpha E	1.11 mg
Saturated Fat	.29 g	Calcium	3.16 mg
Monounsaturated Fat	.5 g	Copper	.04 mg
Polyunsaturated Fat	1.54 g	Iron	.435 mg
Omega 3 Fatty Acid	.077 g	Magnesium	7.69 mg
Omega 6 Fatty Acid	1.45 g	Manganese	.106 mg
Cholesterol	0 mg	Phosphorus	14.6 mg
Dietary Fiber	.659 g	Potassium	72.9 mg
Total Vitamin A	1.34 RE	Selenium	3.15 mcg
A–Retinol	0 RE	Sodium	3.32 mg
A–Carotenoi	1.34 RE	Zinc	.106 mg
Thiamin–B1	.072 mg	Complex Carbohydrates	6.08 g
Riboflavin–B2	.063 mg	Sugars	2.96 g
Niacin–B3	.551 mg	Mono-Saccharide	1.16 g
Niacin Equivalent	.549 mg	Di-Saccharide	1.51 g
Vitamin B6	.091 mg	Alcohol	0 g
Vitamin B12	.004 mcg	Caffeine	0 mg
Folate	5.43 mcg	Water	14.9 g

☉ Cranberry Loaf Cake

Calories	56	Pantothenic	.116 mg
Protein	1.06 g	Vitamin C	.965 mg
Carbohydrates	7.66 g	Vitamin D	0 mcg
Fat—Total	2.46 g	Vitamin E-Alpha E	1.24 mg
Saturated Fat	.285 g	Calcium	5.67 mg
Monounsaturated Fat	.759 g	Copper	.04 mg
Polyunsaturated Fat	1.32 g	Iron	.601 mg
Omega 3 Fatty Acid	.016 g	Magnesium	6.56 mg
Omega 6 Fatty Acid	1.3 g	Manganese	.122 mg
Cholesterol	0 mg	Phosphorus	16.7 mg
Dietary Fiber	.804 g	Potassium	45.2 mg
Total Vitamin A	339 RE	Selenium	2.91 mcg
A–Retinol	0 RE	Sodium	.957 mg
A–Carotenoi	339 RE	Zinc	.135 mg
Thiamin–B1	.074 mg	Complex Carbohydrates	5.96 g
Riboflavin–B2	.049 mg	Sugars	.87 g
Niacin–B3	.528 mg	Mono-Saccharide	.071 g
Niacin Equivalent	.526 mg	Di-Saccharide	.068 g
Vitamin B6	.015 mg	Alcohol	0 g
Vitamin B12	0 mcg	Caffeine	0 mg
Folate	4.32 mcg	Water	16.7 g

⊙ Cream Delight

Calories	25.8	Pantothenic	.003 mg
Protein	.723 g	Vitamin C	.006 mg
Carbohydrates	2.62 g	Vitamin D	.013 mcg
Fat—Total	1.41 g	Vitamin E-Alpha E	.01 mg
Saturated Fat	1.14 g	Calcium	30.5 mg
Monounsaturated Fat	.106 g	Copper	0 mg
Polyunsaturated Fat	.014 g	Iron	.043 mg
Omega 3 Fatty Acid	.005 g	Magnesium	.07 mg
Omega 6 Fatty Acid	.008 g	Manganese	0 mg
Cholesterol	1.74 mg	Phosphorus	.621 mg
Dietary Fiber	0 g	Potassium	.746 mg
Total Vitamin A	4.47 RE	Selenium	.006 mcg
A–Retinol	4.05 RE	Sodium	.373 mg
A–Carotenoi	.119 RE	Zinc	.002 mg
Thiamin–B1	0 mg	Complex Carbohydrates	0 g
Riboflavin–B2	.001 mg	Sugars	1.65 g
Niacin–B3	0 mg	Mono-Saccharide	0 g
Niacin Equivalent	0 mg	Di-Saccharide	.028 g
Vitamin B6	0 mg	Alcohol	0 g
Vitamin B12	.002 mcg	Caffeine	0 mg
Folate	.037 mcg	Water	.572 g

⊙ Creamy Fudge

Calories	19.1	Pantothenic	.014 mg
Protein	.797 g	Vitamin C	.018 mg
Carbohydrates	.668 g	Vitamin D	0 mcg
Fat—Total	1.59 g	Vitamin E-Alpha E	.731 mg
Saturated Fat	.152 g	Calcium	8.11 mg
Monounsaturated Fat	1.03 g	Copper	.029 mg
Polyunsaturated Fat	.335 g	Iron	.112 mg
Omega 3 Fatty Acid	.011 g	Magnesium	9.02 mg
Omega 6 Fatty Acid	.321 g	Manganese	.069 mg
Cholesterol	.234 mg	Phosphorus	15.8 mg
Dietary Fiber	.291 g	Potassium	22.3 mg
Total Vitamin A	3.73 RE	Selenium	.143 mcg
A–Retinol	0 RE	Sodium	8.3 mg
A–Carotenoi	0 RE	Zinc	.089 mg
Thiamin–B1	.006 mg	Complex Carbohydrates	.161 g
Riboflavin–B2	.026 mg	Sugars	.171 g
Niacin–B3	.102 mg	Mono-Saccharide	0 g
Niacin Equivalent	.103 mg	Di-Saccharide	.158 g
Vitamin B6	.003 mg	Alcohol	0 g
Vitamin B12	0 mcg	Caffeine	0 mg
Folate	1.79 mcg	Water	.135 g

⊙ Creamy Strawberries

Calories	58.7	Pantothenic	.014 mg
Protein	2.31 g	Vitamin C	2.35 mg
Carbohydrates	6.66 g	Vitamin D	0 mcg
Fat—Total	2.51 g	Vitamin E-Alpha E	.006 mg
Saturated Fat	2.19 g	Calcium	72.3 mg
Monounsaturated Fat	.002 g	Copper	.002 mg
Polyunsaturated Fat	.008 g	Iron	.119 mg
Omega 3 Fatty Acid	.003 g	Magnesium	.415 mg
Omega 6 Fatty Acid	.004 g	Manganese	.012 mg
Cholesterol	1.66 mg	Phosphorus	.788 mg
Dietary Fiber	.064 g	Potassium	6.9 mg
Total Vitamin A	12.8 RE	Selenium	.037 mcg
A–Retinol	0 RE	Sodium	25.5 mg
A–Carotenoi	.124 RE	Zinc	.005 mg
Thiamin–B1	.001 mg	Complex Carbohydrates	0 g
Riboflavin–B2	.011 mg	Sugars	4.13 g
Niacin–B3	.01 mg	Mono-Saccharide	.195 g
Niacin Equivalent	.01 mg	Di-Saccharide	.046 g
Vitamin B6	.002 mg	Alcohol	0 g
Vitamin B12	0 mcg	Caffeine	0 mg
Folate	.735 mcg	Water	3.8 g

⊙ Crunch Bars

Calories	80.1	Pantothenic	.021 mg
Protein	2.31 g	Vitamin C	0 mg
Carbohydrates	10.3 g	Vitamin D	0 mcg
Fat—Total	3.33 g	Vitamin E-Alpha E	.025 mg
Saturated Fat	2.54 g	Calcium	85.4 mg
Monounsaturated Fat	.306 g	Copper	.009 mg
Polyunsaturated Fat	.088 g	Iron	.37 mg
Omega 3 Fatty Acid	.002 g	Magnesium	1.28 mg
Omega 6 Fatty Acid	.085 g	Manganese	.033 mg
Cholesterol	1.01 mg	Phosphorus	4.98 mg
Dietary Fiber	.128 g	Potassium	34.3 mg
Total Vitamin A	.811 RE	Selenium	.554 mcg
A–Retinol	0 RE	Sodium	30.1 mg
A–Carotenoi	0 RE	Zinc	.037 mg
Thiamin–B1	.027 mg	Complex Carbohydrates	3.18 g
Riboflavin–B2	.022 mg	Sugars	4.41 g
Niacin–B3	.248 mg	Mono-Saccharide	0 g
Niacin Equivalent	.248 mg	Di-Saccharide	0 g
Vitamin B6	.002 mg	Alcohol	0 g
Vitamin B12	0 mcg	Caffeine	0 mg
Folate	1.46 mcg	Water	.194 g

◉ Crunchy Chocolate Cupcakes

Calories	96.7	Pantothenic	.14 mg
Protein	3.3 g	Vitamin C	.102 mg
Carbohydrates	13.5 g	Vitamin D	.354 mcg
Fat—Total	3.4 g	Vitamin E-Alpha E	.739 mg
Saturated Fat	2.05 g	Calcium	98.4 mg
Monounsaturated Fat	.398 g	Copper	.037 mg
Polyunsaturated Fat	.606 g	Iron	.693 mg
Omega 3 Fatty Acid	.029 g	Magnesium	10.5 mg
Omega 6 Fatty Acid	.578 g	Manganese	.471 mg
Cholesterol	.94 mg	Phosphorus	82.2 mg
Dietary Fiber	.721 g	Potassium	108 mg
Total Vitamin A	30.3 RE	Selenium	5.34 mcg
A–Retinol	27.7 RE	Sodium	14.6 mg
A–Carotenoi	1.93 RE	Zinc	.484 mg
Thiamin–B1	.124 mg	Complex Carbohydrates	6.59 g
Riboflavin–B2	.069 mg	Sugars	4.27 g
Niacin–B3	.683 mg	Mono-Saccharide	.071 g
Niacin Equivalent	.684 mg	Di-Saccharide	.761 g
Vitamin B6	.048 mg	Alcohol	0 g
Vitamin B12	.04 mcg	Caffeine	0 mg
Folate	11.4 mcg	Water	12 g

◉ Custard Tarts

Calories	56.9	Pantothenic	.123 mg
Protein	1.52 g	Vitamin C	.528 mg
Carbohydrates	7.63 g	Vitamin D	.529 mcg
Fat—Total	2.27 g	Vitamin E-Alpha E	.35 mg
Saturated Fat	.54 g	Calcium	12.5 mg
Monounsaturated Fat	.806 g	Copper	.015 mg
Polyunsaturated Fat	.728 g	Iron	.41 mg
Omega 3 Fatty Acid	.017 g	Magnesium	3.7 mg
Omega 6 Fatty Acid	.713 g	Manganese	.055 mg
Cholesterol	22.1 mg	Phosphorus	23.2 mg
Dietary Fiber	.355 g	Potassium	46.7 mg
Total Vitamin A	49.4 RE	Selenium	3.82 mcg
A–Retinol	45.6 RE	Sodium	23.6 mg
A–Carotenoi	3.65 RE	Zinc	.13 mg
Thiamin–B1	.056 mg	Complex Carbohydrates	4.46 g
Riboflavin–B2	.07 mg	Sugars	2.67 g
Niacin–B3	.388 mg	Mono-Saccharide	.693 g
Niacin Equivalent	.389 mg	Di-Saccharide	.49 g
Vitamin B6	.02 mg	Alcohol	0 g
Vitamin B12	.074 mcg	Caffeine	0 mg
Folate	4.54 mcg	Water	19.9 g

⊚ Date Balls

Calories	27.5	Pantothenic	.049 mg
Protein	.41 g	Vitamin C	.11 mg
Carbohydrates	2.7 g	Vitamin D	.04 mcg
Fat—Total	1.83 g	Vitamin E-Alpha E	.13 mg
Saturated Fat	.506 g	Calcium	3.05 mg
Monounsaturated Fat	.474 g	Copper	.033 mg
Polyunsaturated Fat	.743 g	Iron	.119 mg
Omega 3 Fatty Acid	.105 g	Magnesium	3.98 mg
Omega 6 Fatty Acid	.629 g	Manganese	.075 mg
Cholesterol	5.33 mg	Phosphorus	9.63 mg
Dietary Fiber	.338 g	Potassium	26.8 mg
Total Vitamin A	8.01 RE	Selenium	.61 mcg
A–Retinol	7.26 RE	Sodium	5.76 mg
A–Carotenoi	.733 RE	Zinc	.083 mg
Thiamin–B1	.012 mg	Complex Carbohydrates	.725 g
Riboflavin–B2	.008 mg	Sugars	1.63 g
Niacin–B3	.12 mg	Mono-Saccharide	.05 g
Niacin Equivalent	.12 mg	Di-Saccharide	1.08 g
Vitamin B6	.016 mg	Alcohol	0 g
Vitamin B12	.015 mcg	Caffeine	0 mg
Folate	2.22 mcg	Water	1.38 g

⊚ Date Cupcakes

Calories	72.1	Pantothenic	.122 mg
Protein	1.51 g	Vitamin C	4.38 mg
Carbohydrates	11.9 g	Vitamin D	.53 mcg
Fat—Total	2.17 g	Vitamin E-Alpha E	.366 mg
Saturated Fat	.392 g	Calcium	14.7 mg
Monounsaturated Fat	.782 g	Copper	.03 mg
Polyunsaturated Fat	.844 g	Iron	.582 mg
Omega 3 Fatty Acid	.014 g	Magnesium	4.88 mg
Omega 6 Fatty Acid	.832 g	Manganese	.085 mg
Cholesterol	8.88 mg	Phosphorus	30.8 mg
Dietary Fiber	.712 g	Potassium	74.6 mg
Total Vitamin A	52.5 RE	Selenium	4.29 mcg
A–Retinol	47 RE	Sodium	19.8 mg
A–Carotenoi	5.35 RE	Zinc	.114 mg
Thiamin–B1	.095 mg	Complex Carbohydrates	7.54 g
Riboflavin–B2	.069 mg	Sugars	3.59 g
Niacin–B3	.722 mg	Mono-Saccharide	.822 g
Niacin Equivalent	.721 mg	Di-Saccharide	1.91 g
Vitamin B6	.02 mg	Alcohol	0 g
Vitamin B12	.023 mcg	Caffeine	0 mg
Folate	7.72 mcg	Water	14.6 g

☺ Date Roll

Calories	34.7	Pantothenic	.046 mg
Protein	.427 g	Vitamin C	.087 mg
Carbohydrates	2.66 g	Vitamin D	.052 mcg
Fat—Total	2.72 g	Vitamin E-Alpha E	.095 mg
Saturated Fat	1.03 g	Calcium	5.4 mg
Monounsaturated Fat	.712 g	Copper	.037 mg
Polyunsaturated Fat	.837 g	Iron	.085 mg
Omega 3 Fatty Acid	.158 g	Magnesium	4.7 mg
Omega 6 Fatty Acid	.67 g	Manganese	.067 mg
Cholesterol	5.43 mg	Phosphorus	10 mg
Dietary Fiber	.314 g	Potassium	32.4 mg
Total Vitamin A	17.1 RE	Selenium	.18 mcg
A–Retinol	16.2 RE	Sodium	1.78 mg
A–Carotenoi	.873 RE	Zinc	.073 mg
Thiamin–B1	.011 mg	Complex Carbohydrates	.233 g
Riboflavin–B2	.01 mg	Sugars	2.1 g
Niacin–B3	.088 mg	Mono-Saccharide	0 g
Niacin Equivalent	.088 mg	Di-Saccharide	1.48 g
Vitamin B6	.018 mg	Alcohol	0 g
Vitamin B12	.007 mcg	Caffeine	0 mg
Folate	1.84 mcg	Water	3.03 g

☺ Dipped Pecans

Calories	55.3	Pantothenic	.048 mg
Protein	1.13 g	Vitamin C	.056 mg
Carbohydrates	3.62 g	Vitamin D	0 mcg
Fat—Total	4.21 g	Vitamin E-Alpha E	.266 mg
Saturated Fat	1.46 g	Calcium	37.1 mg
Monounsaturated Fat	1.66 g	Copper	.032 mg
Polyunsaturated Fat	.805 g	Iron	.109 mg
Omega 3 Fatty Acid	.023 g	Magnesium	3.55 mg
Omega 6 Fatty Acid	.784 g	Manganese	.122 mg
Cholesterol	.454 mg	Phosphorus	8.13 mg
Dietary Fiber	.125 g	Potassium	11.9 mg
Total Vitamin A	14.8 RE	Selenium	.265 mcg
A–Retinol	12.9 RE	Sodium	1.22 mg
A–Carotenoi	1.51 RE	Zinc	.148 mg
Thiamin–B1	.023 mg	Complex Carbohydrates	.25 g
Riboflavin–B2	.007 mg	Sugars	2.08 g
Niacin–B3	.025 mg	Mono-Saccharide	.007 g
Niacin Equivalent	.025 mg	Di-Saccharide	.108 g
Vitamin B6	.005 mg	Alcohol	0 g
Vitamin B12	.002 mcg	Caffeine	0 mg
Folate	1.09 mcg	Water	1.02 g

☺ Dream Balls

Calories	25	Pantothenic	.047 mg
Protein	.381 g	Vitamin C	.237 mg
Carbohydrates	3.59 g	Vitamin D	0 mcg
Fat—Total	1.26 g	Vitamin E-Alpha E	.061 mg
Saturated Fat	.123 g	Calcium	3.21 mg
Monounsaturated Fat	.289 g	Copper	.041 mg
Polyunsaturated Fat	.784 g	Iron	.099 mg
Omega 3 Fatty Acid	.137 g	Magnesium	5.26 mg
Omega 6 Fatty Acid	.638 g	Manganese	.072 mg
Cholesterol	0 mg	Phosphorus	8.22 mg
Dietary Fiber	.414 g	Potassium	42.2 mg
Total Vitamin A	.589 RE	Selenium	.191 mcg
A–Retinol	0 RE	Sodium	.332 mg
A–Carotenoi	.589 RE	Zinc	.069 mg
Thiamin–B1	.012 mg	Complex Carbohydrates	.288 g
Riboflavin–B2	.009 mg	Sugars	2.88 g
Niacin–B3	.114 mg	Mono-Saccharide	.144 g
Niacin Equivalent	.114 mg	Di-Saccharide	1.93 g
Vitamin B6	.029 mg	Alcohol	0 g
Vitamin B12	0 mcg	Caffeine	0 mg
Folate	2.16 mcg	Water	2.33 g

☺ English Toffee

Calories	57.9	Pantothenic	.019 mg
Protein	.942 g	Vitamin C	.025 mg
Carbohydrates	1.52 g	Vitamin D	0 mcg
Fat—Total	5.58 g	Vitamin E-Alpha E	1.4 mg
Saturated Fat	1.09 g	Calcium	19.2 mg
Monounsaturated Fat	2.77 g	Copper	.034 mg
Polyunsaturated Fat	1.46 g	Iron	.143 mg
Omega 3 Fatty Acid	.026 g	Magnesium	10.6 mg
Omega 6 Fatty Acid	1.43 g	Manganese	.08 mg
Cholesterol	.113 mg	Phosphorus	19 mg
Dietary Fiber	.338 g	Potassium	27 mg
Total Vitamin A	42.4 RE	Selenium	.167 mcg
A–Retinol	38.7 RE	Sodium	.484 mg
A–Carotenoi	3.48 RE	Zinc	.104 mg
Thiamin–B1	.008 mg	Complex Carbohydrates	.188 g
Riboflavin–B2	.029 mg	Sugars	.708 g
Niacin–B3	.12 mg	Mono-Saccharide	0 g
Niacin Equivalent	.12 mg	Di-Saccharide	.185 g
Vitamin B6	.004 mg	Alcohol	0 g
Vitamin B12	.002 mcg	Caffeine	0 mg
Folate	2.11 mcg	Water	.945 g

⊘ Fancy Pecans

Calories	34.2	Pantothenic	.065 mg
Protein	.381 g	Vitamin C	.129 mg
Carbohydrates	6.53 g	Vitamin D	0 mcg
Fat—Total	1.11 g	Vitamin E-Alpha E	.075 mg
Saturated Fat	.101 g	Calcium	10.5 mg
Monounsaturated Fat	.656 g	Copper	.046 mg
Polyunsaturated Fat	.288 g	Iron	.217 mg
Omega 3 Fatty Acid	.011 g	Magnesium	6.52 mg
Omega 6 Fatty Acid	.278 g	Manganese	.101 mg
Cholesterol	0 mg	Phosphorus	10.6 mg
Dietary Fiber	.799 g	Potassium	70.2 mg
Total Vitamin A	1.09 RE	Selenium	.571 mcg
A–Retinol	0 RE	Sodium	.908 mg
A–Carotenoi	1.09 RE	Zinc	.122 mg
Thiamin–B1	.021 mg	Complex Carbohydrates	.14 g
Riboflavin–B2	.01 mg	Sugars	5.6 g
Niacin–B3	.101 mg	Mono-Saccharide	4.54 g
Niacin Equivalent	.101 mg	Di-Saccharide	1.13 g
Vitamin B6	.023 mg	Alcohol	0 g
Vitamin B12	0 mcg	Caffeine	0 mg
Folate	1.29 mcg	Water	2.36 g

⊘ Fig Sticks

Calories	59.1	Pantothenic	.077 mg
Protein	1.49 g	Vitamin C	.11 mg
Carbohydrates	8.24 g	Vitamin D	0 mcg
Fat—Total	2.86 g	Vitamin E-Alpha E	.856 mg
Saturated Fat	.332 g	Calcium	27.4 mg
Monounsaturated Fat	1.52 g	Copper	.093 mg
Polyunsaturated Fat	.871 g	Iron	.52 mg
Omega 3 Fatty Acid	.02 g	Magnesium	22.8 mg
Omega 6 Fatty Acid	.849 g	Manganese	.145 mg
Cholesterol	0 mg	Phosphorus	39.2 mg
Dietary Fiber	1.54 g	Potassium	112 mg
Total Vitamin A	1.63 RE	Selenium	.982 mcg
A–Retinol	0 RE	Sodium	2.36 mg
A–Carotenoi	1.63 RE	Zinc	.347 mg
Thiamin–B1	.028 mg	Complex Carbohydrates	.199 g
Riboflavin–B2	.037 mg	Sugars	6.57 g
Niacin–B3	.276 mg	Mono-Saccharide	6.67 g
Niacin Equivalent	.276 mg	Di-Saccharide	.909 g
Vitamin B6	.032 mg	Alcohol	0 g
Vitamin B12	0 mcg	Caffeine	0 mg
Folate	4.56 mcg	Water	3.46 g

⊚ Filled Fruit

Calories	53.1	Pantothenic	.064 mg
Protein	1.39 g	Vitamin C	2.59 mg
Carbohydrates	3.15 g	Vitamin D	0 mcg
Fat—Total	3.9 g	Vitamin E-Alpha E	.837 mg
Saturated Fat	.717 g	Calcium	4.47 mg
Monounsaturated Fat	1.78 g	Copper	.023 mg
Polyunsaturated Fat	1.2 g	Iron	.14 mg
Omega 3 Fatty Acid	.014 g	Magnesium	2.14 mg
Omega 6 Fatty Acid	1.19 g	Manganese	.02 mg
Cholesterol	1.25 mg	Phosphorus	5.55 mg
Dietary Fiber	.465 g	Potassium	77.7 mg
Total Vitamin A	134 RE	Selenium	.337 mcg
A–Retinol	43 RE	Sodium	42.8 mg
A–Carotenoi	71.4 RE	Zinc	.067 mg
Thiamin–B1	.008 mg	Complex Carbohydrates	0 g
Riboflavin–B2	.026 mg	Sugars	2.28 g
Niacin–B3	.156 mg	Mono-Saccharide	.595 g
Niacin Equivalent	.156 mg	Di-Saccharide	1.6 g
Vitamin B6	.014 mg	Alcohol	0 g
Vitamin B12	.003 mcg	Caffeine	0 mg
Folate	2.25 mcg	Water	23.4 g

⊚ Friendly Dates

Calories	57.8	Pantothenic	.078 mg
Protein	1.09 g	Vitamin C	.74 mg
Carbohydrates	5.24 g	Vitamin D	0 mcg
Fat—Total	4.14 g	Vitamin E-Alpha E	.185 mg
Saturated Fat	.382 g	Calcium	11.6 mg
Monounsaturated Fat	.95 g	Copper	.109 mg
Polyunsaturated Fat	2.61 g	Iron	.26 mg
Omega 3 Fatty Acid	.451 g	Magnesium	13.9 mg
Omega 6 Fatty Acid	2.12 g	Manganese	.211 mg
Cholesterol	0 mg	Phosphorus	24.1 mg
Dietary Fiber	.785 g	Potassium	72.9 mg
Total Vitamin A	1.43 RE	Selenium	.556 mcg
A–Retinol	0 RE	Sodium	1.07 mg
A–Carotenoi	1.43 RE	Zinc	.205 mg
Thiamin–B1	.03 mg	Complex Carbohydrates	.815 g
Riboflavin–B2	.015 mg	Sugars	3.64 g
Niacin–B3	.153 mg	Mono-Saccharide	1.68 g
Niacin Equivalent	.151 mg	Di-Saccharide	1.59 g
Vitamin B6	.049 mg	Alcohol	0 g
Vitamin B12	0 mcg	Caffeine	0 mg
Folate	5.06 mcg	Water	2.29 g

☺ Frosted Fruit

Calories	3.7	Pantothenic	.036 mg
Protein	.203 g	Vitamin C	5.71 mg
Carbohydrates	.721 g	Vitamin D	0 mcg
Fat—Total	.037 g	Vitamin E-Alpha E	.014 mg
Saturated Fat	.002 g	Calcium	1.5 mg
Monounsaturated Fat	.005 g	Copper	.005 mg
Polyunsaturated Fat	.019 g	Iron	.039 mg
Omega 3 Fatty Acid	.008 g	Magnesium	1.16 mg
Omega 6 Fatty Acid	.011 g	Manganese	.029 mg
Cholesterol	0 mg	Phosphorus	2.09 mg
Dietary Fiber	.154 g	Potassium	18.7 mg
Total Vitamin A	.302 RE	Selenium	.328 mcg
A–Retinol	0 RE	Sodium	2.32 mg
A–Carotenoi	.302 RE	Zinc	.013 mg
Thiamin–B1	.002 mg	Complex Carbohydrates	0 g
Riboflavin–B2	.013 mg	Sugars	.582 g
Niacin–B3	.024 mg	Mono-Saccharide	.488 g
Niacin Equivalent	.024 mg	Di-Saccharide	.111 g
Vitamin B6	.006 mg	Alcohol	0 g
Vitamin B12	.003 mcg	Caffeine	0 mg
Folate	1.83 mcg	Water	10.4 g

☺ Frozen Fruit

Calories	41	Pantothenic	.086 mg
Protein	.79 g	Vitamin C	2.88 mg
Carbohydrates	6.01 g	Vitamin D	.157 mcg
Fat—Total	1.75 g	Vitamin E-Alpha E	.047 mg
Saturated Fat	1.41 g	Calcium	25.2 mg
Monounsaturated Fat	.144 g	Copper	.027 mg
Polyunsaturated Fat	.079 g	Iron	.113 mg
Omega 3 Fatty Acid	.025 g	Magnesium	5.05 mg
Omega 6 Fatty Acid	.034 g	Manganese	.289 mg
Cholesterol	.283 mg	Phosphorus	17.7 mg
Dietary Fiber	.254 g	Potassium	52.7 mg
Total Vitamin A	16.6 RE	Selenium	.276 mcg
A–Retinol	9.2 RE	Sodium	11.5 mg
A–Carotenoi	7.39 RE	Zinc	.091 mg
Thiamin–B1	.02 mg	Complex Carbohydrates	.205 g
Riboflavin–B2	.033 mg	Sugars	5.56 g
Niacin–B3	.097 mg	Mono-Saccharide	.861 g
Niacin Equivalent	.086 mg	Di-Saccharide	1.43 g
Vitamin B6	.022 mg	Alcohol	0 g
Vitamin B12	.019 mcg	Caffeine	0 mg
Folate	2.81 mcg	Water	30.5 g

⊙ Fruit Bars

Calories	66.5	Pantothenic	.167 mg
Protein	.968 g	Vitamin C	.293 mg
Carbohydrates	10.6 g	Vitamin D	0 mcg
Fat—Total	2.92 g	Vitamin E-Alpha E	.764 mg
Saturated Fat	.897 g	Calcium	15.5 mg
Monounsaturated Fat	.5 g	Copper	.104 mg
Polyunsaturated Fat	1.36 g	Iron	.444 mg
Omega 3 Fatty Acid	.156 g	Magnesium	12.4 mg
Omega 6 Fatty Acid	1.19 g	Manganese	.171 mg
Cholesterol	0 mg	Phosphorus	31.5 mg
Dietary Fiber	1.45 g	Potassium	120 mg
Total Vitamin A	1.49 RE	Selenium	2.1 mcg
A–Retinol	0 RE	Sodium	1.95 mg
A–Carotenoi	1.49 RE	Zinc	.202 mg
Thiamin–B1	.026 mg	Complex Carbohydrates	.385 g
Riboflavin–B2	.02 mg	Sugars	8.75 g
Niacin–B3	.25 mg	Mono-Saccharide	5.55 g
Niacin Equivalent	.249 mg	Di-Saccharide	2.52 g
Vitamin B6	.053 mg	Alcohol	0 g
Vitamin B12	0 mcg	Caffeine	0 mg
Folate	5.95 mcg	Water	4.47 g

⊙ Fruit Crêpes

Calories	58.3	Pantothenic	.249 mg
Protein	2.32 g	Vitamin C	2.81 mg
Carbohydrates	8.14 g	Vitamin D	.366 mcg
Fat—Total	2.1 g	Vitamin E-Alpha E	.4 mg
Saturated Fat	.838 g	Calcium	33.5 mg
Monounsaturated Fat	.68 g	Copper	.023 mg
Polyunsaturated Fat	.244 g	Iron	.273 mg
Omega 3 Fatty Acid	.028 g	Magnesium	6.28 mg
Omega 6 Fatty Acid	.216 g	Manganese	.025 mg
Cholesterol	56 mg	Phosphorus	44.5 mg
Dietary Fiber	.907 g	Potassium	99 mg
Total Vitamin A	32.6 RE	Selenium	4.39 mcg
A–Retinol	29.4 RE	Sodium	25.8 mg
A–Carotenoi	3.05 RE	Zinc	.234 mg
Thiamin–B1	.023 mg	Complex Carbohydrates	.005 g
Riboflavin–B2	.103 mg	Sugars	6.64 g
Niacin–B3	.062 mg	Mono-Saccharide	3.99 g
Niacin Equivalent	.062 mg	Di-Saccharide	2.15 g
Vitamin B6	.048 mg	Alcohol	0 g
Vitamin B12	.198 mcg	Caffeine	0 mg
Folate	8.18 mcg	Water	65.9 g

⊙ Fruit Surprise

Calories	26.2	Pantothenic	.01 mg
Protein	.643 g	Vitamin C	.052 mg
Carbohydrates	2.11 g	Vitamin D	.019 mcg
Fat—Total	1.77 g	Vitamin E-Alpha E	.217 mg
Saturated Fat	1.08 g	Calcium	21.2 mg
Monounsaturated Fat	.443 g	Copper	.011 mg
Polyunsaturated Fat	.113 g	Iron	.072 mg
Omega 3 Fatty Acid	.011 g	Magnesium	3.01 mg
Omega 6 Fatty Acid	.101 g	Manganese	.028 mg
Cholesterol	2.26 mg	Phosphorus	5.95 mg
Dietary Fiber	.148 g	Potassium	13.5 mg
Total Vitamin A	6.53 RE	Selenium	.154 mcg
A–Retinol	6.08 RE	Sodium	.758 mg
A–Carotenoi	.274 RE	Zinc	.035 mg
Thiamin–B1	.003 mg	Complex Carbohydrates	.111 g
Riboflavin–B2	.009 mg	Sugars	1.28 g
Niacin–B3	.039 mg	Mono-Saccharide	.017 g
Niacin Equivalent	.039 mg	Di-Saccharide	.084 g
Vitamin B6	.003 mg	Alcohol	0 g
Vitamin B12	.003 mcg	Caffeine	0 mg
Folate	.789 mcg	Water	1.14 g

⊙ Graham Cracker Crust

Calories	70.4	Pantothenic	.067 mg
Protein	.856 g	Vitamin C	.006 mg
Carbohydrates	9.24 g	Vitamin D	.604 mcg
Fat—Total	3.41 g	Vitamin E-Alpha E	.424 mg
Saturated Fat	.666 g	Calcium	3.89 mg
Monounsaturated Fat	1.43 g	Copper	.024 mg
Polyunsaturated Fat	1.11 g	Iron	.449 mg
Omega 3 Fatty Acid	.019 g	Magnesium	3.69 mg
Omega 6 Fatty Acid	1.09 g	Manganese	.097 mg
Cholesterol	0 mg	Phosphorus	13.3 mg
Dietary Fiber	.324 g	Potassium	17.6 mg
Total Vitamin A	56.4 RE	Selenium	1.32 mcg
A–Retinol	51.6 RE	Sodium	92.6 mg
A–Carotenoi	4.64 RE	Zinc	.097 mg
Thiamin–B1	.027 mg	Complex Carbohydrates	3.23 g
Riboflavin–B2	.039 mg	Sugars	5.68 g
Niacin–B3	.495 mg	Mono-Saccharide	0 g
Niacin Equivalent	.495 mg	Di-Saccharide	0 g
Vitamin B6	.008 mg	Alcohol	0 g
Vitamin B12	.003 mcg	Caffeine	0 mg
Folate	2.08 mcg	Water	3.83 g

☉ Granola Candy

Calories	29.9	Pantothenic	.033 mg
Protein	.653 g	Vitamin C	.078 mg
Carbohydrates	3.5 g	Vitamin D	0 mcg
Fat—Total	1.66 g	Vitamin E-Alpha E	.244 mg
Saturated Fat	.492 g	Calcium	3.34 mg
Monounsaturated Fat	.403 g	Copper	.033 mg
Polyunsaturated Fat	.72 g	Iron	.223 mg
Omega 3 Fatty Acid	.034 g	Magnesium	6.18 mg
Omega 6 Fatty Acid	.682 g	Manganese	.012 mg
Cholesterol	0 mg	Phosphorus	21.7 mg
Dietary Fiber	.612 g	Potassium	28.5 mg
Total Vitamin A	.178 RE	Selenium	1.18 mcg
A–Retinol	0 RE	Sodium	5.01 mg
A–Carotenoi	.178 RE	Zinc	.196 mg
Thiamin–B1	.031 mg	Complex Carbohydrates	.879 g
Riboflavin–B2	.013 mg	Sugars	1.44 g
Niacin–B3	.094 mg	Mono-Saccharide	.508 g
Niacin Equivalent	.094 mg	Di-Saccharide	.909 g
Vitamin B6	.018 mg	Alcohol	0 g
Vitamin B12	0 mcg	Caffeine	0 mg
Folate	4.34 mcg	Water	1.61 g

☉ Granola Delight

Calories	31.3	Pantothenic	.04 mg
Protein	.358 g	Vitamin C	.065 mg
Carbohydrates	3.97 g	Vitamin D	0 mcg
Fat—Total	1.77 g	Vitamin E-Alpha E	.229 mg
Saturated Fat	.642 g	Calcium	2.62 mg
Monounsaturated Fat	.527 g	Copper	.026 mg
Polyunsaturated Fat	.529 g	Iron	.148 mg
Omega 3 Fatty Acid	.016 g	Magnesium	3.85 mg
Omega 6 Fatty Acid	.511 g	Manganese	.029 mg
Cholesterol	0 mg	Phosphorus	11.2 mg
Dietary Fiber	.562 g	Potassium	34.6 mg
Total Vitamin A	9.62 RE	Selenium	.726 mcg
A–Retinol	8.6 RE	Sodium	4.05 mg
A–Carotenoi	.993 RE	Zinc	.098 mg
Thiamin–B1	.016 mg	Complex Carbohydrates	.352 g
Riboflavin–B2	.009 mg	Sugars	2.59 g
Niacin–B3	.109 mg	Mono-Saccharide	.237 g
Niacin Equivalent	.109 mg	Di-Saccharide	1.69 g
Vitamin B6	.014 mg	Alcohol	0 g
Vitamin B12	.001 mcg	Caffeine	0 mg
Folate	2.38 mcg	Water	2.38 g

☺ Happy Trails

Calories	85.6	Pantothenic	.054 mg
Protein	2.59 g	Vitamin C	.083 mg
Carbohydrates	9.48 g	Vitamin D	.035 mcg
Fat—Total	4.38 g	Vitamin E-Alpha E	.33 mg
Saturated Fat	2.39 g	Calcium	71.3 mg
Monounsaturated Fat	.756 g	Copper	.038 mg
Polyunsaturated Fat	.879 g	Iron	.332 mg
Omega 3 Fatty Acid	.029 g	Magnesium	8.44 mg
Omega 6 Fatty Acid	.845 g	Manganese	.049 mg
Cholesterol	.854 mg	Phosphorus	24.7 mg
Dietary Fiber	.582 g	Potassium	33.8 mg
Total Vitamin A	.837 RE	Selenium	1.14 mcg
A–Retinol	0 RE	Sodium	7.81 mg
A–Carotenoi	.151 RE	Zinc	.231 mg
Thiamin–B1	.037 mg	Complex Carbohydrates	1.69 g
Riboflavin–B2	.013 mg	Sugars	5.02 g
Niacin–B3	.378 mg	Mono-Saccharide	.421 g
Niacin Equivalent	.378 mg	Di-Saccharide	.913 g
Vitamin B6	.021 mg	Alcohol	0 g
Vitamin B12	.003 mcg	Caffeine	0 mg
Folate	6.09 mcg	Water	.224 g

☺ Haupia

Calories	7.51	Pantothenic	.015 mg
Protein	.387 g	Vitamin C	.058 mg
Carbohydrates	.228 g	Vitamin D	.031 mcg
Fat—Total	.607 g	Vitamin E-Alpha E	.018 mg
Saturated Fat	.538 g	Calcium	4.42 mg
Monounsaturated Fat	.027 g	Copper	.012 mg
Polyunsaturated Fat	.007 g	Iron	.098 mg
Omega 3 Fatty Acid	0 g	Magnesium	1.71 mg
Omega 6 Fatty Acid	.007 g	Manganese	.022 mg
Cholesterol	.055 mg	Phosphorus	5.9 mg
Dietary Fiber	.032 g	Potassium	11.3 mg
Total Vitamin A	1.86 RE	Selenium	.235 mcg
A–Retinol	1.86 RE	Sodium	2.46 mg
A–Carotenoi	0 RE	Zinc	.028 mg
Thiamin–B1	.002 mg	Complex Carbohydrates	0 g
Riboflavin–B2	.005 mg	Sugars	.197 g
Niacin–B3	.021 mg	Mono-Saccharide	0 g
Niacin Equivalent	.021 mg	Di-Saccharide	.149 g
Vitamin B6	.002 mg	Alcohol	0 g
Vitamin B12	.012 mcg	Caffeine	0 mg
Folate	.619 mcg	Water	4.88 g

⊚ Heavenly Puffs

Calories	102	Pantothenic	.129 mg
Protein	2.51 g	Vitamin C	.043 mg
Carbohydrates	16 g	Vitamin D	.727 mcg
Fat—Total	3.01 g	Vitamin E-Alpha E	.504 mg
Saturated Fat	.537 g	Calcium	7.25 mg
Monounsaturated Fat	1.07 g	Copper	.031 mg
Polyunsaturated Fat	1.18 g	Iron	1.05 mg
Omega 3 Fatty Acid	.02 g	Magnesium	4.98 mg
Omega 6 Fatty Acid	1.16 g	Manganese	.163 mg
Cholesterol	12.2 mg	Phosphorus	28.2 mg
Dietary Fiber	.743 g	Potassium	59.2 mg
Total Vitamin A	69.9 RE	Selenium	7.87 mcg
A–Retinol	64.4 RE	Sodium	62.9 mg
A–Carotenoi	5.34 RE	Zinc	.179 mg
Thiamin–B1	.163 mg	Complex Carbohydrates	14.8 g
Riboflavin–B2	.118 mg	Sugars	.428 g
Niacin–B3	1.22 mg	Mono-Saccharide	.221 g
Niacin Equivalent	1.22 mg	Di-Saccharide	.082 g
Vitamin B6	.015 mg	Alcohol	0 g
Vitamin B12	.032 mcg	Caffeine	0 mg
Folate	6.73 mcg	Water	8.38 g

⊚ Lemon Biscotti

Calories	69.3	Pantothenic	.101 mg
Protein	2.03 g	Vitamin C	.451 mg
Carbohydrates	6.88 g	Vitamin D	.241 mcg
Fat—Total	4.2 g	Vitamin E-Alpha E	.388 mg
Saturated Fat	.681 g	Calcium	15 mg
Monounsaturated Fat	1.79 g	Copper	.07 mg
Polyunsaturated Fat	1.47 g	Iron	.627 mg
Omega 3 Fatty Acid	.041 g	Magnesium	13.5 mg
Omega 6 Fatty Acid	1.43 g	Manganese	.221 mg
Cholesterol	13.1 mg	Phosphorus	37.9 mg
Dietary Fiber	.836 g	Potassium	76.7 mg
Total Vitamin A	25.2 RE	Selenium	3.77 mcg
A–Retinol	23.1 RE	Sodium	15.4 mg
A–Carotenoi	2.04 RE	Zinc	.272 mg
Thiamin–B1	.12 mg	Complex Carbohydrates	5.6 g
Riboflavin–B2	.068 mg	Sugars	.437 g
Niacin–B3	.617 mg	Mono-Saccharide	.119 g
Niacin Equivalent	.617 mg	Di-Saccharide	.053 g
Vitamin B6	.016 mg	Alcohol	0 g
Vitamin B12	.034 mcg	Caffeine	0 mg
Folate	6.56 mcg	Water	5.68 g

❂ Lemon Cheesecake

Calories	121	Pantothenic	.446 mg
Protein	4.73 g	Vitamin C	1.39 mg
Carbohydrates	17.9 g	Vitamin D	1.62 mcg
Fat—Total	3.54 g	Vitamin E-Alpha E	.43 mg
Saturated Fat	.731 g	Calcium	152 mg
Monounsaturated Fat	1.46 g	Copper	.033 mg
Polyunsaturated Fat	1.12 g	Iron	.608 mg
Omega 3 Fatty Acid	.021 g	Magnesium	17.6 mg
Omega 6 Fatty Acid	1.1 g	Manganese	.1 mg
Cholesterol	1.84 mg	Phosphorus	134 mg
Dietary Fiber	.364 g	Potassium	189 mg
Total Vitamin A	116 RE	Selenium	2.66 mcg
A–Retinol	111 RE	Sodium	189 mg
A–Carotenoi	4.68 RE	Zinc	.559 mg
Thiamin–B1	.051 mg	Complex Carbohydrates	3.23 g
Riboflavin–B2	.197 mg	Sugars	11.6 g
Niacin–B3	.585 mg	Mono-Saccharide	.027 g
Niacin Equivalent	.585 mg	Di-Saccharide	5.83 g
Vitamin B6	.037 mg	Alcohol	0 g
Vitamin B12	.125 mcg	Caffeine	0 mg
Folate	6.61 mcg	Water	45.6 g

❂ Lemon Squares

Calories	33.4	Pantothenic	.035 mg
Protein	.719 g	Vitamin C	.178 mg
Carbohydrates	4.82 g	Vitamin D	.308 mcg
Fat—Total	1.21 g	Vitamin E-Alpha E	.204 mg
Saturated Fat	.206 g	Calcium	1.7 mg
Monounsaturated Fat	.435 g	Copper	.009 mg
Polyunsaturated Fat	.494 g	Iron	.297 mg
Omega 3 Fatty Acid	.007 g	Magnesium	1.49 mg
Omega 6 Fatty Acid	.489 g	Manganese	.043 mg
Cholesterol	1.96 mg	Phosphorus	7.99 mg
Dietary Fiber	.206 g	Potassium	8.45 mg
Total Vitamin A	29.1 RE	Selenium	2.26 mcg
A–Retinol	26.7 RE	Sodium	10.7 mg
A–Carotenoi	2.33 RE	Zinc	.049 mg
Thiamin–B1	.05 mg	Complex Carbohydrates	4.46 g
Riboflavin–B2	.034 mg	Sugars	.157 g
Niacin–B3	.37 mg	Mono-Saccharide	.07 g
Niacin Equivalent	.37 mg	Di-Saccharide	.026 g
Vitamin B6	.004 mg	Alcohol	0 g
Vitamin B12	.006 mcg	Caffeine	0 mg
Folate	1.91 mcg	Water	3.12 g

⊚ Maple Bars

Calories	17.3	Pantothenic	.024 mg
Protein	.45 g	Vitamin C	.001 mg
Carbohydrates	2.66 g	Vitamin D	.121 mcg
Fat—Total	.512 g	Vitamin E-Alpha E	.084 mg
Saturated Fat	.094 g	Calcium	1.05 mg
Monounsaturated Fat	.182 g	Copper	.005 mg
Polyunsaturated Fat	.195 g	Iron	.171 mg
Omega 3 Fatty Acid	.003 g	Magnesium	.85 mg
Omega 6 Fatty Acid	.192 g	Manganese	.024 mg
Cholesterol	2.96 mg	Phosphorus	5.13 mg
Dietary Fiber	.114 g	Potassium	4.83 mg
Total Vitamin A	11.8 RE	Selenium	1.39 mcg
A–Retinol	10.9 RE	Sodium	17.8 mg
A–Carotenoi	.859 RE	Zinc	.032 mg
Thiamin–B1	.028 mg	Complex Carbohydrates	2.48 g
Riboflavin–B2	.021 mg	Sugars	.072 g
Niacin–B3	.206 mg	Mono-Saccharide	.04 g
Niacin Equivalent	.206 mg	Di-Saccharide	.014 g
Vitamin B6	.003 mg	Alcohol	0 g
Vitamin B12	.008 mcg	Caffeine	0 mg
Folate	1.24 mcg	Water	1.55 g

⊚ Maple Pudding

Calories	100	Pantothenic	.325 mg
Protein	3.98 g	Vitamin C	.716 mg
Carbohydrates	6.15 g	Vitamin D	.062 mcg
Fat—Total	7.12 g	Vitamin E-Alpha E	.273 mg
Saturated Fat	1.35 g	Calcium	96.3 mg
Monounsaturated Fat	1.51 g	Copper	.15 mg
Polyunsaturated Fat	3.93 g	Iron	.301 mg
Omega 3 Fatty Acid	.688 g	Magnesium	25.8 mg
Omega 6 Fatty Acid	3.19 g	Manganese	.317 mg
Cholesterol	1.05 mg	Phosphorus	104 mg
Dietary Fiber	.456 g	Potassium	166 mg
Total Vitamin A	7.17 RE	Selenium	1.99 mcg
A–Retinol	3.12 RE	Sodium	41.7 mg
A–Carotenoi	4.04 RE	Zinc	.692 mg
Thiamin–B1	.06 mg	Complex Carbohydrates	1.41 g
Riboflavin–B2	.118 mg	Sugars	4.28 g
Niacin–B3	.16 mg	Mono-Saccharide	0 g
Niacin Equivalent	.16 mg	Di-Saccharide	.21 g
Vitamin B6	.079 mg	Alcohol	0 g
Vitamin B12	.265 mcg	Caffeine	.229 mg
Folate	11.8 mcg	Water	40.5 g

⊚ Mock Chocolate Cake

Calories	54.9	Pantothenic	.078 mg
Protein	1.24 g	Vitamin C	.017 mg
Carbohydrates	6.47 g	Vitamin D	.07 mcg
Fat—Total	2.66 g	Vitamin E-Alpha E	1.41 mg
Saturated Fat	.375 g	Calcium	21.2 mg
Monounsaturated Fat	.599 g	Copper	.017 mg
Polyunsaturated Fat	1.57 g	Iron	.417 mg
Omega 3 Fatty Acid	.013 g	Magnesium	2.78 mg
Omega 6 Fatty Acid	1.56 g	Manganese	.054 mg
Cholesterol	13.4 mg	Phosphorus	34.8 mg
Dietary Fiber	.651 g	Potassium	51.6 mg
Total Vitamin A	7.87 RE	Selenium	3.44 mcg
A–Retinol	7.85 RE	Sodium	6.15 mg
A–Carotenoi	.013 RE	Zinc	.106 mg
Thiamin–B1	.057 mg	Complex Carbohydrates	5 g
Riboflavin–B2	.059 mg	Sugars	.294 g
Niacin–B3	.429 mg	Mono-Saccharide	.1 g
Niacin Equivalent	.429 mg	Di-Saccharide	.166 g
Vitamin B6	.012 mg	Alcohol	0 g
Vitamin B12	.042 mcg	Caffeine	0 mg
Folate	3.69 mcg	Water	3.23 g

⊚ Nut Crunch

Calories	35.3	Pantothenic	.012 mg
Protein	.594 g	Vitamin C	.037 mg
Carbohydrates	1.12 g	Vitamin D	0 mcg
Fat—Total	3.32 g	Vitamin E-Alpha E	.554 mg
Saturated Fat	.654 g	Calcium	12.6 mg
Monounsaturated Fat	1.48 g	Copper	.029 mg
Polyunsaturated Fat	1.02 g	Iron	.093 mg
Omega 3 Fatty Acid	.064 g	Magnesium	6.55 mg
Omega 6 Fatty Acid	.948 g	Manganese	.059 mg
Cholesterol	.085 mg	Phosphorus	12 mg
Dietary Fiber	.204 g	Potassium	17.4 mg
Total Vitamin A	21.3 RE	Selenium	.12 mcg
A–Retinol	19.3 RE	Sodium	.315 mg
A–Carotenoi	1.83 RE	Zinc	.089 mg
Thiamin–B1	.006 mg	Complex Carbohydrates	.201 g
Riboflavin–B2	.014 mg	Sugars	.499 g
Niacin–B3	.062 mg	Mono-Saccharide	0 g
Niacin Equivalent	.062 mg	Di-Saccharide	.107 g
Vitamin B6	.006 mg	Alcohol	0 g
Vitamin B12	.001 mcg	Caffeine	0 mg
Folate	1.58 mcg	Water	.487 g

⊚ Oatmeal Cookies

Calories	45.8	Pantothenic	.047 mg
Protein	.665 g	Vitamin C	.014 mg
Carbohydrates	3.29 g	Vitamin D	.015 mcg
Fat—Total	3.4 g	Vitamin E-Alpha E	1.59 mg
Saturated Fat	.886 g	Calcium	4.54 mg
Monounsaturated Fat	.63 g	Copper	.015 mg
Polyunsaturated Fat	1.77 g	Iron	.226 mg
Omega 3 Fatty Acid	.013 g	Magnesium	2.96 mg
Omega 6 Fatty Acid	1.76 g	Manganese	.079 mg
Cholesterol	5.07 mg	Phosphorus	13.2 mg
Dietary Fiber	.352 g	Potassium	15.6 mg
Total Vitamin A	2.36 RE	Selenium	1.99 mcg
A–Retinol	2.27 RE	Sodium	18 mg
A–Carotenoi	.089 RE	Zinc	.08 mg
Thiamin–B1	.031 mg	Complex Carbohydrates	2.62 g
Riboflavin–B2	.023 mg	Sugars	.322 g
Niacin–B3	.189 mg	Mono-Saccharide	.042 g
Niacin Equivalent	.19 mg	Di-Saccharide	.034 g
Vitamin B6	.007 mg	Alcohol	0 g
Vitamin B12	.012 mcg	Caffeine	0 mg
Folate	1.64 mcg	Water	6.04 g

⊚ Old-Fashioned Candy Canes

Calories	.053	Pantothenic	0 mg
Protein	0 g	Vitamin C	0 mg
Carbohydrates	.014 g	Vitamin D	0 mcg
Fat—Total	0 g	Vitamin E-Alpha E	0 mg
Saturated Fat	0 g	Calcium	.012 mg
Monounsaturated Fat	0 g	Copper	0 mg
Polyunsaturated Fat	0 g	Iron	0 mg
Omega 3 Fatty Acid	0 g	Magnesium	.006 mg
Omega 6 Fatty Acid	0 g	Manganese	0 mg
Cholesterol	0 mg	Phosphorus	0 mg
Dietary Fiber	0 g	Potassium	.653 mg
Total Vitamin A	0 RE	Selenium	0 mcg
A–Retinol	0 RE	Sodium	.076 mg
A–Carotenoi	0 RE	Zinc	0 mg
Thiamin–B1	0 mg	Complex Carbohydrates	0 g
Riboflavin–B2	0 mg	Sugars	.014 g
Niacin–B3	0 mg	Mono-Saccharide	0 g
Niacin Equivalent	0 mg	Di-Saccharide	0 g
Vitamin B6	0 mg	Alcohol	0 g
Vitamin B12	0 mcg	Caffeine	0 mg
Folate	0 mcg	Water	.615 g

❂ Orange Pound Cake

Calories	82.9	Pantothenic	.196 mg
Protein	2.67 g	Vitamin C	.006 mg
Carbohydrates	9.61 g	Vitamin D	.861 mcg
Fat—Total	3.68 g	Vitamin E-Alpha E	.536 mg
Saturated Fat	.767 g	Calcium	23.9 mg
Monounsaturated Fat	1.35 g	Copper	.019 mg
Polyunsaturated Fat	1.23 g	Iron	.754 mg
Omega 3 Fatty Acid	.023 g	Magnesium	3.99 mg
Omega 6 Fatty Acid	1.21 g	Manganese	.087 mg
Cholesterol	47.3 mg	Phosphorus	58.4 mg
Dietary Fiber	.398 g	Potassium	64.2 mg
Total Vitamin A	83.9 RE	Selenium	7.54 mcg
A–Retinol	78.6 RE	Sodium	36.8 mg
A–Carotenoi	5.16 RE	Zinc	.211 mg
Thiamin–B1	.103 mg	Complex Carbohydrates	8.83 g
Riboflavin–B2	.118 mg	Sugars	.37 g
Niacin–B3	.727 mg	Mono-Saccharide	.247 g
Niacin Equivalent	.727 mg	Di-Saccharide	.040 g
Vitamin B6	.021 mg	Alcohol	0 g
Vitamin B12	.115 mcg	Caffeine	0 mg
Folate	8.43 mcg	Water	13.5 g

❂ Orange Sticks

Calories	24.3	Pantothenic	.04 mg
Protein	.44 g	Vitamin C	.655 mg
Carbohydrates	2.04 g	Vitamin D	0 mcg
Fat—Total	1.76 g	Vitamin E-Alpha E	.177 mg
Saturated Fat	.442 g	Calcium	11 mg
Monounsaturated Fat	.546 g	Copper	.028 mg
Polyunsaturated Fat	.683 g	Iron	.121 mg
Omega 3 Fatty Acid	.077 g	Magnesium	4.39 mg
Omega 6 Fatty Acid	.602 g	Manganese	.064 mg
Cholesterol	.048 mg	Phosphorus	17.3 mg
Dietary Fiber	.219 g	Potassium	37.5 mg
Total Vitamin A	12.6 RE	Selenium	.422 mcg
A–Retinol	9.17 RE	Sodium	4.37 mg
A–Carotenoi	1.23 RE	Zinc	.073 mg
Thiamin–B1	.012 mg	Complex Carbohydrates	.325 g
Riboflavin–B2	.012 mg	Sugars	1.16 g
Niacin–B3	.04 mg	Mono-Saccharide	.926 g
Niacin Equivalent	.033 mg	Di-Saccharide	.073 g
Vitamin B6	.012 mg	Alcohol	0 g
Vitamin B12	.012 mcg	Caffeine	.632 mg
Folate	1.48 mcg	Water	1.79 g

⊚ Peach Pie

Calories	52	Pantothenic	.159 mg
Protcin	.935 g	Vitamin C	5.83 mg
Carbohydrates	12.2 g	Vitamin D	0 mcg
Fat—Total	.425 g	Vitamin E-Alpha E	.609 mg
Saturated Fat	.287 g	Calcium	4.83 mg
Monounsaturated Fat	.052 g	Copper	.063 mg
Polyunsaturated Fat	.058 g	Iron	.24 mg
Omega 3 Fatty Acid	.005 g	Magnesium	6.69 mg
Omega 6 Fatty Acid	.054 g	Manganese	.062 mg
Cholesterol	0 mg	Phosphorus	13.7 mg
Dietary Fiber	1.63 g	Potassium	172 mg
Total Vitamin A	46.6 RE	Sclenium	2.17 mcg
A–Retinol	0 RE	Sodium	.384 mg
A–Carotenoi	46.6 RE	Zinc	.142 mg
Thiamin–B1	.039 mg	Complex Carbohydrates	2.23 g
Riboflavin–B2	.051 mg	Sugars	7.88 g
Niacin–B3	1.03 mg	Mono-Saccharide	2.08 g
Niacin Equivalent	1.02 mg	Di-Saccharide	5.36 g
Vitamin B6	.017 mg	Alcohol	0 g
Vitamin B12	0 mcg	Caffeine	.632 mg
Folate	3.77 mcg	Water	76 g

⊚ Peach Tarts

Calories	54.4	Pantothenic	.07 mg
Protein	.819 g	Vitamin C	1.34 mg
Carbohydrates	9.45 g	Vitamin D	.403 mcg
Fat—Total	1.56 g	Vitamin E-Alpha E	.393 mg
Saturated Fat	.256 g	Calcium	3.3 mg
Monounsaturated Fat	.562 g	Copper	.024 mg
Polyunsaturated Fat	.655 g	Iron	.349 mg
Omega 3 Fatty Acid	.01 g	Magnesium	3.41 mg
Omega 6 Fatty Acid	.647 g	Manganese	.06 mg
Cholesterol	0 mg	Phosphorus	10.6 mg
Dietary Fiber	.574 g	Potassium	61.1 mg
Total Vitamin A	47.9 RE	Selenium	2.39 mcg
A–Retinol	34.4 RE	Sodium	14.4 mg
A–Carotenoi	13.3 RE	Zinc	.076 mg
Thiamin–B1	.053 mg	Complex Carbohydrates	5.54 g
Riboflavin–B2	.041 mg	Sugars	3.18 g
Niacin–B3	.563 mg	Mono-Saccharide	.516 g
Niacin Equivalent	.563 mg	Di-Saccharide	1.23 g
Vitamin B6	.011 mg	Alcohol	0 g
Vitamin B12	.002 mcg	Caffeine	0 mg
Folate	2.34 mcg	Water	21.8 g

⊚ Peach Upside-Down Cake

Calories	23.9	Pantothenic	.054 mg
Protein	.752 g	Vitamin C	.785 mg
Carbohydrates	4.16 g	Vitamin D	.02 mcg
Fat—Total	.476 g	Vitamin E-Alpha E	.297 mg
Saturated Fat	.06 g	Calcium	7.29 mg
Monounsaturated Fat	.096 g	Copper	.011 mg
Polyunsaturated Fat	.302 g	Iron	.29 mg
Omega 3 Fatty Acid	.003 g	Magnesium	1.93 mg
Omega 6 Fatty Acid	.295 g	Manganese	.031 mg
Cholesterol	.069 mg	Phosphorus	9.3 mg
Dietary Fiber	.259 g	Potassium	27.6 mg
Total Vitamin A	4.18 RE	Selenium	.729 mcg
A–Retinol	1.2 RE	Sodium	5.98 mg
A–Carotenoi	2.98 RE	Zinc	.061 mg
Thiamin–B1	.037 mg	Complex Carbohydrates	2.8 g
Riboflavin–B2	.036 mg	Sugars	1.05 g
Niacin–B3	.316 mg	Mono-Saccharide	.149 g
Niacin Equivalent	.313 mg	Di-Saccharide	.427 g
Vitamin B6	.006 mg	Alcohol	0 g
Vitamin B12	.023 mcg	Caffeine	0 mg
Folate	1.34 mcg	Water	12.9 g

⊚ Peanut Butter Balls

Calories	16.4	Pantothenic	.028 mg
Protein	.451 g	Vitamin C	.066 mg
Carbohydrates	.649 g	Vitamin D	0 mcg
Fat—Total	1.47 g	Vitamin E-Alpha E	.135 mg
Saturated Fat	.705 g	Calcium	1.15 mg
Monounsaturated Fat	.424 g	Copper	.019 mg
Polyunsaturated Fat	.258 g	Iron	.085 mg
Omega 3 Fatty Acid	0 g	Magnesium	3.46 mg
Omega 6 Fatty Acid	.258 g	Manganese	.063 mg
Cholesterol	0 mg	Phosphorus	8.01 mg
Dietary Fiber	.294 g	Potassium	17.7 mg
Total Vitamin A	0 RE	Selenium	.513 mcg
A–Retinol	0 RE	Sodium	.496 mg
A–Carotenoi	0 RE	Zinc	.075 mg
Thiamin–B1	.008 mg	Complex Carbohydrates	.118 g
Riboflavin–B2	.002 mg	Sugars	.244 g
Niacin–B3	.227 mg	Mono-Saccharide	.068 g
Niacin Equivalent	.227 mg	Di-Saccharide	.002 g
Vitamin B6	.007 mg	Alcohol	0 g
Vitamin B12	0 mcg	Caffeine	0 mg
Folate	2.85 mcg	Water	.964 g

☺ Peanut Butter and Banana Fudge

Calories	14.2	Pantothenic	.034 mg
Protein	.545 g	Vitamin C	.325 mg
Carbohydrates	1.15 g	Vitamin D	0 mcg
Fat—Total	.942 g	Vitamin E-Alpha E	.005 mg
Saturated Fat	.174 g	Calcium	.929 mg
Monounsaturated Fat	.42 g	Copper	.018 mg
Polyunsaturated Fat	.258 g	Iron	.047 mg
Omega 3 Fatty Acid	.002 g	Magnesium	4.13 mg
Omega 6 Fatty Acid	.256 g	Manganese	.034 mg
Cholesterol	0 mg	Phosphorus	7.64 mg
Dietary Fiber	.18 g	Potassium	26.7 mg
Total Vitamin A	.094 RE	Selenium	.035 mcg
A–Retinol	0 RE	Sodium	.462 mg
A–Carotenoi	.094 RE	Zinc	.063 mg
Thiamin–B1	.006 mg	Complex Carbohydrates	.652 g
Riboflavin–B2	.004 mg	Sugars	.385 g
Niacin–B3	.297 mg	Mono-Saccharide	.11 g
Niacin Equivalent	.297 mg	Di-Saccharide	.239 g
Vitamin B6	.023 mg	Alcohol	0 g
Vitamin B12	0 mcg	Caffeine	0 mg
Folate	1.88 mcg	Water	3.18 g

☺ Peanut Butter Bars

Calories	77.5	Pantothenic	.154 mg
Protein	2.56 g	Vitamin C	.001 mg
Carbohydrates	6.7 g	Vitamin D	.036 mcg
Fat—Total	4.75 g	Vitamin E-Alpha E	.719 mg
Saturated Fat	.769 g	Calcium	6.08 mg
Monounsaturated Fat	2.25 g	Copper	.053 mg
Polyunsaturated Fat	1.45 g	Iron	.505 mg
Omega 3 Fatty Acid	.009 g	Magnesium	12.9 mg
Omega 6 Fatty Acid	1.44 g	Manganese	.179 mg
Cholesterol	11.8 mg	Phosphorus	35.2 mg
Dietary Fiber	.663 g	Potassium	52.7 mg
Total Vitamin A	21 RE	Selenium	3.68 mcg
A–Retinol	19.6 RE	Sodium	4.05 mg
A–Carotenoi	1.29 RE	Zinc	.288 mg
Thiamin–B1	.084 mg	Complex Carbohydrates	5.58 g
Riboflavin–B2	.055 mg	Sugars	.45 g
Niacin–B3	1.26 mg	Mono-Saccharide	.11 g
Niacin Equivalent	1.26 mg	Di-Saccharide	.28 g
Vitamin B6	.023 mg	Alcohol	0 g
Vitamin B12	.029 mcg	Caffeine	0 mg
Folate	12.3 mcg	Water	3.31 g

☺ Peanut Butter Cookies

Calories	53.1	Pantothenic	.138 mg
Protein	2.26 g	Vitamin C	0 mg
Carbohydrates	1.97 g	Vitamin D	.019 mcg
Fat—Total	4.43 g	Vitamin E-Alpha E	.653 mg
Saturated Fat	.673 g	Calcium	6.69 mg
Monounsaturated Fat	2.16 g	Copper	.058 mg
Polyunsaturated Fat	1.36 g	Iron	.216 mg
Omega 3 Fatty Acid	.001 g	Magnesium	15.2 mg
Omega 6 Fatty Acid	1.36 g	Manganese	.178 mg
Cholesterol	6.25 mg	Phosphorus	33.3 mg
Dietary Fiber	.563 g	Potassium	58 mg
Total Vitamin A	2.81 RE	Selenium	1.09 mcg
A–Retinol	2.8 RE	Sodium	2.36 mg
A–Carotenoi	0 RE	Zinc	.299 mg
Thiamin–B1	.038 mg	Complex Carbohydrates	.632 g
Riboflavin–B2	.017 mg	Sugars	.732 g
Niacin–B3	1.15 mg	Mono-Saccharide	.018 g
Niacin Equivalent	1.15 mg	Di-Saccharide	0 g
Vitamin B6	.036 mg	Alcohol	0 g
Vitamin B12	.015 mcg	Caffeine	0 mg
Folate	13.1 mcg	Water	1.23 g

☺ Peanut Butter and Cream Cheese Kisses

Calories	36	Pantothenic	.031 mg
Protein	1.79 g	Vitamin C	0 mg
Carbohydrates	2.4 g	Vitamin D	0 mcg
Fat—Total	2.21 g	Vitamin E-Alpha E	.24 mg
Saturated Fat	.854 g	Calcium	19.3 mg
Monounsaturated Fat	.755 g	Copper	.017 mg
Polyunsaturated Fat	.461 g	Iron	.087 mg
Omega 3 Fatty Acid	.002 g	Magnesium	5.09 mg
Omega 6 Fatty Acid	.458 g	Manganese	.059 mg
Cholesterol	.975 mg	Phosphorus	10.1 mg
Dietary Fiber	.212 g	Potassium	23.9 mg
Total Vitamin A	12.1 RE	Selenium	.24 mcg
A–Retinol	0 RE	Sodium	26 mg
A–Carotenoi	0 RE	Zinc	.089 mg
Thiamin–B1	.004 mg	Complex Carbohydrates	.221 g
Riboflavin–B2	.012 mg	Sugars	1.23 g
Niacin–B3	.438 mg	Mono-Saccharide	.038 g
Niacin Equivalent	.438 mg	Di-Saccharide	.212 g
Vitamin B6	.014 mg	Alcohol	0 g
Vitamin B12	0 mcg	Caffeine	0 mg
Folate	2.94 mcg	Water	.036 g

⊚ Peanut Butter Cups

Calories	91.9	Pantothenic	.059 mg
Protein	3.42 g	Vitamin C	0 mg
Carbohydrates	7.25 g	Vitamin D	0 mcg
Fat—Total	5.85 g	Vitamin E-Alpha E	0 mg
Saturated Fat	2.81 g	Calcium	74 mg
Monounsaturated Fat	1.51 g	Copper	.042 mg
Polyunsaturated Fat	.922 g	Iron	.224 mg
Omega 3 Fatty Acid	.005 g	Magnesium	11.5 mg
Omega 6 Fatty Acid	.916 g	Manganese	.102 mg
Cholesterol	.907 mg	Phosphorus	22.4 mg
Dietary Fiber	.422 g	Potassium	44.4 mg
Total Vitamin A	.73 RE	Selenium	0 mcg
A–Retinol	0 RE	Sodium	1.09 mg
A–Carotenoi	0 RE	Zinc	.192 mg
Thiamin–B1	.01 mg	Complex Carbohydrates	.398 g
Riboflavin–B2	.006 mg	Sugars	4.4 g
Niacin–B3	.908 mg	Mono-Saccharide	.077 g
Niacin Equivalent	.908 mg	Di-Saccharide	.422 g
Vitamin B6	.028 mg	Alcohol	0 g
Vitamin B12	0 mcg	Caffeine	0 mg
Folate	5 mcg	Water	.077 g

⊚ Peanut Butter Fudge

Calories	10.9	Pantothenic	.031 mg
Protein	.414 g	Vitamin C	.131 mg
Carbohydrates	.698 g	Vitamin D	0 mcg
Fat—Total	.797 g	Vitamin E-Alpha E	.121 mg
Saturated Fat	.11 g	Calcium	1.01 mg
Monounsaturated Fat	.395 g	Copper	.014 mg
Polyunsaturated Fat	.252 g	Iron	.042 mg
Omega 3 Fatty Acid	0 g	Magnesium	3.17 mg
Omega 6 Fatty Acid	.252 g	Manganese	.036 mg
Cholesterol	0 mg	Phosphorus	6.46 mg
Dietary Fiber	.129 g	Potassium	16.4 mg
Total Vitamin A	0 RE	Selenium	.133 mcg
A–Retinol	0 RE	Sodium	.185 mg
A–Carotenoi	0 RE	Zinc	.058 mg
Thiamin–B1	.009 mg	Complex Carbohydrates	.423 g
Riboflavin–B2	.002 mg	Sugars	.138 g
Niacin–B3	.239 mg	Mono-Saccharide	0 g
Niacin Equivalent	.239 mg	Di-Saccharide	0 g
Vitamin B6	.011 mg	Alcohol	0 g
Vitamin B12	0 mcg	Caffeine	0 mg
Folate	2.48 mcg	Water	1.4 g

⊚ Peanut Butter-Potato Pinwheels

Calories	21.7	Pantothenic	.042 mg
Protein	.85 g	Vitamin C	.133 mg
Carbohydrates	1.1 g	Vitamin D	0 mcg
Fat—Total	1.7 g	Vitamin E-Alpha E	.257 mg
Saturated Fat	.327 g	Calcium	1.55 mg
Monounsaturated Fat	.805 g	Copper	.021 mg
Polyunsaturated Fat	.493 g	Iron	.07 mg
Omega 3 Fatty Acid	.003 g	Magnesium	5.79 mg
Omega 6 Fatty Acid	.489 g	Manganese	.066 mg
Cholesterol	0 mg	Phosphorus	11.5 mg
Dietary Fiber	.25 g	Potassium	33.1 mg
Total Vitamin A	0 RE	Selenium	.27 mcg
A–Retinol	0 RE	Sodium	.671 mg
A–Carotenoi	0 RE	Zinc	.1 mg
Thiamin–B1	.006 mg	Complex Carbohydrates	.545 g
Riboflavin–B2	.004 mg	Sugars	.295 g
Niacin–B3	.491 mg	Mono-Saccharide	.041 g
Niacin Equivalent	.491 mg	Di-Saccharide	.226 g
Vitamin B6	.02 mg	Alcohol	0 g
Vitamin B12	0 mcg	Caffeine	0 mg
Folate	3.3 mcg	Water	1.45 g

⊚ Pie Crust

Calories	68.2	Pantothenic	.055 mg
Protein	1.29 g	Vitamin C	0 mg
Carbohydrates	9.54 g	Vitamin D	0 mcg
Fat—Total	2.69 g	Vitamin E-Alpha E	.423 mg
Saturated Fat	.661 g	Calcium	1.88 mg
Monounsaturated Fat	1.15 g	Copper	.018 mg
Polyunsaturated Fat	.72 g	Iron	.581 mg
Omega 3 Fatty Acid	.044 g	Magnesium	2.75 mg
Omega 6 Fatty Acid	.676 g	Manganese	.086 mg
Cholesterol	0 mg	Phosphorus	13.5 mg
Dietary Fiber	.409 g	Potassium	13.4 mg
Total Vitamin A	0 RE	Selenium	4.24 mcg
A–Retinol	0 RE	Sodium	.25 mg
A–Carotenoi	0 RE	Zinc	.088 mg
Thiamin–B1	.098 mg	Complex Carbohydrates	8.91 g
Riboflavin–B2	.062 mg	Sugars	.213 g
Niacin–B3	.738 mg	Mono-Saccharide	.113 g
Niacin Equivalent	.738 mg	Di-Saccharide	.05 g
Vitamin B6	.006 mg	Alcohol	0 g
Vitamin B12	0 mcg	Caffeine	0 mg
Folate	3.25 mcg	Water	1.49 g

⊚ Pineapple Pie

Calories	92.8	Pantothenic	.176 mg
Protein	1.69 g	Vitamin C	2.62 mg
Carbohydrates	12.4 g	Vitamin D	.064 mcg
Fat—Total	4.21 g	Vitamin E-Alpha E	.168 mg
Saturated Fat	2.13 g	Calcium	32.2 mg
Monounsaturated Fat	1.46 g	Copper	.047 mg
Polyunsaturated Fat	.317 g	Iron	.533 mg
Omega 3 Fatty Acid	.059 g	Magnesium	8.81 mg
Omega 6 Fatty Acid	.255 g	Manganese	.366 mg
Cholesterol	9.44 mg	Phosphorus	40.9 mg
Dietary Fiber	.512 g	Potassium	71.5 mg
Total Vitamin A	28.7 RE	Selenium	1.62 mcg
A–Retinol	25.4 RE	Sodium	87.7 mg
A–Carotenoi	3.29 RE	Zinc	.242 mg
Thiamin–B1	.05 mg	Complex Carbohydrates	3.38 g
Riboflavin–B2	.083 mg	Sugars	8.55 g
Niacin–B3	.578 mg	Mono-Saccharide	.775 g
Niacin Equivalent	.578 mg	Di-Saccharide	1.51 g
Vitamin B6	.026 mg	Alcohol	0 g
Vitamin B12	.081 mcg	Caffeine	.137 mg
Folate	6.4 mcg	Water	35.4 g

⊚ Potato Bon Bons

Calories	27.3	Pantothenic	.055 mg
Protein	.748 g	Vitamin C	.799 mg
Carbohydrates	4.24 g	Vitamin D	0 mcg
Fat—Total	.842 g	Vitamin E-Alpha E	.005 mg
Saturated Fat	.734 g	Calcium	24.8 mg
Monounsaturated Fat	0 g	Copper	.018 mg
Polyunsaturated Fat	.005 g	Iron	.068 mg
Omega 3 Fatty Acid	.001 g	Magnesium	2.16 mg
Omega 6 Fatty Acid	.004 g	Manganese	.015 mg
Cholesterol	.302 mg	Phosphorus	4.32 mg
Dietary Fiber	.141 g	Potassium	35.4 mg
Total Vitamin A	.243 RE	Selenium	.086 mcg
A–Retinol	0 RE	Sodium	.541 mg
A–Carotenoi	0 RE	Zinc	.029 mg
Thiamin–B1	.011 mg	Complex Carbohydrates	1.86 g
Riboflavin–B2	.002 mg	Sugars	1.41 g
Niacin–B3	.142 mg	Mono-Saccharide	0 g
Niacin Equivalent	.142 mg	Di-Saccharide	0 g
Vitamin B6	.029 mg	Alcohol	0 g
Vitamin B12	0 mcg	Caffeine	0 mg
Folate	.96 mcg	Water	8.4 g

☻ Pralines

Calories	39.2	Pantothenic	.099 mg
Protein	.531 g	Vitamin C	.142 mg
Carbohydrates	1.13 g	Vitamin D	.002 mcg
Fat—Total	3.89 g	Vitamin E-Alpha E	.22 mg
Saturated Fat	.368 g	Calcium	6.38 mg
Monounsaturated Fat	2.36 g	Copper	.061 mg
Polyunsaturated Fat	.976 g	Iron	.113 mg
Omega 3 Fatty Acid	.037 g	Magnesium	7.04 mg
Omega 6 Fatty Acid	.939 g	Manganese	.234 mg
Cholesterol	.134 mg	Phosphorus	18.5 mg
Dietary Fiber	.24 g	Potassium	26.2 mg
Total Vitamin A	5.37 RE	Selenium	.346 mcg
A–Retinol	4.3 RE	Sodium	23.7 mg
A–Carotenoi	1.06 RE	Zinc	.3 mg
Thiamin–B1	.045 mg	Complex Carbohydrates	.479 g
Riboflavin–B2	.013 mg	Sugars	.409 g
Niacin–B3	.048 mg	Mono-Saccharide	.008 g
Niacin Equivalent	.048 mg	Di-Saccharide	.349 g
Vitamin B6	.011 mg	Alcohol	0 g
Vitamin B12	.009 mcg	Caffeine	0 mg
Folate	2.22 mcg	Water	3.78 g

☻ Pretzels

Calories	71.6	Pantothenic	0 mg
Protein	2.25 g	Vitamin C	0 mg
Carbohydrates	8.3 g	Vitamin D	0 mcg
Fat—Total	3.33 g	Vitamin E-Alpha E	0 mg
Saturated Fat	2.92 g	Calcium	95.7 mg
Monounsaturated Fat	0 g	Copper	0 mg
Polyunsaturated Fat	0 g	Iron	.137 mg
Omega 3 Fatty Acid	0 g	Magnesium	0 mg
Omega 6 Fatty Acid	0 g	Manganese	0 mg
Cholesterol	1.21 mg	Phosphorus	0 mg
Dietary Fiber	0 g	Potassium	0 mg
Total Vitamin A	.973 RE	Selenium	0 mcg
A–Retinol	0 RE	Sodium	0 mg
A–Carotenoi	0 RE	Zinc	0 mg
Thiamin–B1	0 mg	Complex Carbohydrates	0 g
Riboflavin–B2	0 mg	Sugars	5.2 g
Niacin–B3	0 mg	Mono-Saccharide	0 g
Niacin Equivalent	0 mg	Di-Saccharide	0 g
Vitamin B6	0 mg	Alcohol	0 g
Vitamin B12	0 mcg	Caffeine	0 mg
Folate	0 mcg	Water	0 g

☺ Prune Purée

Calories	454	Pantothenic	.789 mg
Protein	4.45 g	Vitamin C	5.61 mg
Carbohydrates	119 g	Vitamin D	0 mcg
Fat—Total	.885 g	Vitamin E-Alpha E	2.27 mg
Saturated Fat	.069 g	Calcium	87 mg
Monounsaturated Fat	.579 g	Copper	.732 mg
Polyunsaturated Fat	.19 g	Iron	4.24 mg
Omega 3 Fatty Acid	0 g	Magnesium	76.5 mg
Omega 6 Fatty Acid	.19 g	Manganese	.4 mg
Cholesterol	0 mg	Phosphorus	147 mg
Dietary Fiber	15.7 g	Potassium	1269 mg
Total Vitamin A	338 RE	Selenium	4.45 mcg
A–Retinol	0 RE	Sodium	63.5 mg
A–Carotenoi	338 RE	Zinc	.907 mg
Thiamin–B1	.141 mg	Complex Carbohydrates	0 g
Riboflavin–B2	.278 mg	Sugars	73.1 g
Niacin–B3	3.35 mg	Mono-Saccharide	63.2 g
Niacin Equivalent	3.35 mg	Di-Saccharide	1.36 g
Vitamin B6	.45 mg	Alcohol	0 g
Vitamin B12	0 mcg	Caffeine	0 mg
Folate	6.3 mcg	Water	70.7 g

☺ Pumpkin Pie

Calories	58.1	Pantothenic	.559 mg
Protein	3.29 g	Vitamin C	2.23 mg
Carbohydrates	7.03 g	Vitamin D	.694 mcg
Fat—Total	2.11 g	Vitamin E-Alpha E	.629 mg
Saturated Fat	.916 g	Calcium	92.7 mg
Monounsaturated Fat	.64 g	Copper	.054 mg
Polyunsaturated Fat	.225 g	Iron	.882 mg
Omega 3 Fatty Acid	.019 g	Magnesium	17.8 mg
Omega 6 Fatty Acid	.207 g	Manganese	.073 mg
Cholesterol	64.8 mg	Phosphorus	90 mg
Dietary Fiber	1.27 g	Potassium	183 mg
Total Vitamin A	1061 RE	Selenium	3.45 mcg
A–Retinol	58.9 RE	Sodium	34.1 mg
A–Carotenoi	1002 RE	Zinc	.463 mg
Thiamin–B1	.031 mg	Complex Carbohydrates	.904 g
Riboflavin–B2	.135 mg	Sugars	4.86 g
Niacin–B3	.211 mg	Mono-Saccharide	.089 g
Niacin Equivalent	.212 mg	Di-Saccharide	2.91 g
Vitamin B6	.059 mg	Alcohol	0 g
Vitamin B12	.216 mcg	Caffeine	0 mg
Folate	15 mcg	Water	64.3 g

⊚ Pumpkin Squares

Calories	1.57	Pantothenic	.006 mg
Protein	.172 g	Vitamin C	.145 mg
Carbohydrates	.191 g	Vitamin D	0 mcg
Fat—Total	.003 g	Vitamin E-Alpha E	.022 mg
Saturated Fat	.001 g	Calcium	.504 mg
Monounsaturated Fat	0 g	Copper	.003 mg
Polyunsaturated Fat	0 g	Iron	.019 mg
Omega 3 Fatty Acid	0 g	Magnesium	.284 mg
Omega 6 Fatty Acid	0 g	Manganese	.004 mg
Cholesterol	.187 mg	Phosphorus	.926 mg
Dietary Fiber	.028 g	Potassium	7.09 mg
Total Vitamin A	36.1 RE	Selenium	.031 mcg
A–Retinol	0 RE	Sodium	6.4 mg
A–Carotenoi	33.1 RE	Zinc	.007 mg
Thiamin–B1	.001 mg	Complex Carbohydrates	.002 g
Riboflavin–B2	.005 mg	Sugars	.1 g
Niacin–B3	.013 mg	Mono-Saccharide	.068 g
Niacin Equivalent	.013 mg	Di-Saccharide	.03 g
Vitamin B6	.001 mg	Alcohol	0 g
Vitamin B12	0 mcg	Caffeine	0 mg
Folate	.26 mcg	Water	2.87 g

⊚ Pumpkin Tarts

Calories	12.3	Pantothenic	.077 mg
Protein	.75 g	Vitamin C	.316 mg
Carbohydrates	.973 g	Vitamin D	.094 mcg
Fat—Total	.63 g	Vitamin E-Alpha E	.093 mg
Saturated Fat	.35 g	Calcium	10.2 mg
Monounsaturated Fat	.167 g	Copper	.008 mg
Polyunsaturated Fat	.046 g	Iron	.126 mg
Omega 3 Fatty Acid	.007 g	Magnesium	2.66 mg
Omega 6 Fatty Acid	.039 g	Manganese	.01 mg
Cholesterol	11.5 mg	Phosphorus	12.6 mg
Dietary Fiber	.172 g	Potassium	27.2 mg
Total Vitamin A	143 RE	Selenium	1.24 mcg
A–Retinol	6.42 RE	Sodium	9.11 mg
A–Carotenoi	136 RE	Zinc	.062 mg
Thiamin–B1	.005 mg	Complex Carbohydrates	.122 g
Riboflavin–B2	.033 mg	Sugars	.679 g
Niacin–B3	.031 mg	Mono-Saccharide	.047 g
Niacin Equivalent	.031 mg	Di-Saccharide	.285 g
Vitamin B6	.01 mg	Alcohol	0 g
Vitamin B12	.05 mcg	Caffeine	0 mg
Folate	2.28 mcg	Water	14.4 g

⊚ Raisin Clusters

Calories	35.9	Pantothenic	.001 mg
Protein	1 g	Vitamin C	.067 mg
Carbohydrates	5.05 g	Vitamin D	0 mcg
Fat—Total	1.4 g	Vitamin E-Alpha E	.014 mg
Saturated Fat	1.22 g	Calcium	40.8 mg
Monounsaturated Fat	0 g	Copper	.006 mg
Polyunsaturated Fat	.003 g	Iron	.099 mg
Omega 3 Fatty Acid	.001 g	Magnesium	.665 mg
Omega 6 Fatty Acid	.002 g	Manganese	.006 mg
Cholesterol	.504 mg	Phosphorus	1.96 mg
Dietary Fiber	.07 g	Potassium	15.1 mg
Total Vitamin A	.421 RE	Selenium	.134 mcg
A–Retinol	0 RE	Sodium	.242 mg
A–Carotenoi	.016 RE	Zinc	.005 mg
Thiamin–B1	.003 mg	Complex Carbohydrates	0 g
Riboflavin–B2	.002 mg	Sugars	3.68 g
Niacin–B3	.017 mg	Mono-Saccharide	1.31 g
Niacin Equivalent	.017 mg	Di-Saccharide	0 g
Vitamin B6	.005 mg	Alcohol	0 g
Vitamin B12	0 mcg	Caffeine	0 mg
Folate	.067 mcg	Water	.31 g

⊚ Rascal Raspberries

Calories	49.2	Pantothenic	.007 mg
Protein	1.52 g	Vitamin C	.684 mg
Carbohydrates	5.85 g	Vitamin D	0 mcg
Fat—Total	2.23 g	Vitamin E-Alpha E	.012 mg
Saturated Fat	1.95 g	Calcium	64.4 mg
Monounsaturated Fat	.001 g	Copper	.002 mg
Polyunsaturated Fat	.009 g	Iron	.107 mg
Omega 3 Fatty Acid	.003 g	Magnesium	.491 mg
Omega 6 Fatty Acid	.006 g	Manganese	.028 mg
Cholesterol	.806 mg	Phosphorus	.329 mg
Dietary Fiber	.108 g	Potassium	4.16 mg
Total Vitamin A	1 RE	Selenium	.014 mcg
A–Retinol	0 RE	Sodium	.001 mg
A–Carotenoi	.356 RE	Zinc	.013 mg
Thiamin–B1	.001 mg	Complex Carbohydrates	0 g
Riboflavin–B2	.002 mg	Sugars	3.73 g
Niacin–B3	.025 mg	Mono-Saccharide	.183 g
Niacin Equivalent	0 mg	Di-Saccharide	.076 g
Vitamin B6	.002 mg	Alcohol	0 g
Vitamin B12	0 mcg	Caffeine	0 mg
Folate	.711 mcg	Water	2.4 g

⊚ Raspberry Crunch

Calories	55.9	Pantothenic	.092 mg
Protein	1.06 g	Vitamin C	.365 mg
Carbohydrates	5.24 g	Vitamin D	.53 mcg
Fat—Total	3.45 g	Vitamin E-Alpha E	.401 mg
Saturated Fat	.484 g	Calcium	3.86 mg
Monounsaturated Fat	1.61 g	Copper	.033 mg
Polyunsaturated Fat	1.16 g	Iron	.359 mg
Omega 3 Fatty Acid	.027 g	Magnesium	4.42 mg
Omega 6 Fatty Acid	1.13 g	Manganese	.143 mg
Cholesterol	8.88 mg	Phosphorus	16.7 mg
Dietary Fiber	.339 g	Potassium	25 mg
Total Vitamin A	51.4 RE	Selenium	2.78 mcg
A–Retinol	47 RE	Sodium	20 mg
A–Carotenoi	4.29 RE	Zinc	.181 mg
Thiamin–B1	.066 mg	Complex Carbohydrates	4.45 g
Riboflavin–B2	.045 mg	Sugars	.467 g
Niacin–B3	.385 mg	Mono-Saccharide	.166 g
Niacin Equivalent	.374 mg	Di-Saccharide	.139 g
Vitamin B6	.01 mg	Alcohol	0 g
Vitamin B12	.023 mcg	Caffeine	0 mg
Folate	3.68 mcg	Water	11.2 g

⊚ Spice Delight

Calories	38.5	Pantothenic	.035 mg
Protein	.728 g	Vitamin C	.018 mg
Carbohydrates	4.84 g	Vitamin D	.459 mcg
Fat—Total	1.77 g	Vitamin E-Alpha E	.291 mg
Saturated Fat	.305 g	Calcium	2.38 mg
Monounsaturated Fat	.643 g	Copper	.01 mg
Polyunsaturated Fat	.726 g	Iron	.311 mg
Omega 3 Fatty Acid	.01 g	Magnesium	1.6 mg
Omega 6 Fatty Acid	.718 g	Manganese	.053 mg
Cholesterol	1.96 mg	Phosphorus	8.26 mg
Dietary Fiber	.23 g	Potassium	8.81 mg
Total Vitamin A	43.2 RE	Selenium	2.27 mcg
A–Retinol	39.6 RE	Sodium	15.7 mg
A–Carotenoi	3.5 RE	Zinc	.051 mg
Thiamin–B1	.05 mg	Complex Carbohydrates	4.47 g
Riboflavin–B2	.034 mg	Sugars	.143 g
Niacin–B3	.371 mg	Mono-Saccharide	.062 g
Niacin Equivalent	.371 mg	Di-Saccharide	.025 g
Vitamin B6	.004 mg	Alcohol	0 g
Vitamin B12	.007 mcg	Caffeine	0 mg
Folate	1.87 mcg	Water	3.61 g

⊚ Striped Candy Canes

Calories	5.08	Pantothenic	.012 mg
Protein	1.06 g	Vitamin C	0 mg
Carbohydrates	.105 g	Vitamin D	0 mcg
Fat—Total	0 g	Vitamin E-Alpha E	0 mg
Saturated Fat	0 g	Calcium	.608 mg
Monounsaturated Fat	0 g	Copper	.001 mg
Polyunsaturated Fat	0 g	Iron	.003 mg
Omega 3 Fatty Acid	0 g	Magnesium	1.11 mg
Omega 6 Fatty Acid	0 g	Manganese	0 mg
Cholesterol	0 mg	Phosphorus	1.32 mg
Dietary Fiber	0 g	Potassium	14.5 mg
Total Vitamin A	0 RE	Selenium	1.78 mcg
A–Retinol	0 RE	Sodium	16.6 mg
A–Carotenoi	0 RE	Zinc	.001 mg
Thiamin–B1	.001 mg	Complex Carbohydrates	0 g
Riboflavin–B2	.046 mg	Sugars	.105 g
Niacin–B3	.009 mg	Mono-Saccharide	.105 g
Niacin Equivalent	.009 mg	Di-Saccharide	0 g
Vitamin B6	0 mg	Alcohol	0 g
Vitamin B12	.02 mcg	Caffeine	0 mg
Folate	.304 mcg	Water	8.89 g

⊚ Stuffed Dates

Calories	42	Pantothenic	.113 mg
Protein	.603 g	Vitamin C	.025 mg
Carbohydrates	7.46 g	Vitamin D	0 mcg
Fat—Total	1.54 g	Vitamin E-Alpha E	.148 mg
Saturated Fat	.177 g	Calcium	4.2 mg
Monounsaturated Fat	.865 g	Copper	.051 mg
Polyunsaturated Fat	.419 g	Iron	.166 mg
Omega 3 Fatty Acid	.008 g	Magnesium	7.24 mg
Omega 6 Fatty Acid	.407 g	Manganese	.112 mg
Cholesterol	0 mg	Phosphorus	12.2 mg
Dietary Fiber	.855 g	Potassium	75.2 mg
Total Vitamin A	.631 RE	Selenium	.343 mcg
A–Retinol	0 RE	Sodium	.376 mg
A–Carotenoi	.631 RE	Zinc	.14 mg
Thiamin–B1	.025 mg	Complex Carbohydrates	.213 g
Riboflavin–B2	.012 mg	Sugars	6.39 g
Niacin–B3	.399 mg	Mono-Saccharide	0 g
Niacin Equivalent	.399 mg	Di-Saccharide	4.26 g
Vitamin B6	.026 mg	Alcohol	0 g
Vitamin B12	0 mcg	Caffeine	0 mg
Folate	3.61 mcg	Water	2.21 g

☻ Sweet Almonds

Calories	26.3	Pantothenic	.017 mg
Protein	.744 g	Vitamin C	.022 mg
Carbohydrates	.674 g	Vitamin D	0 mcg
Fat—Total	2.47 g	Vitamin E-Alpha E	.294 mg
Saturated Fat	.287 g	Calcium	9.07 mg
Monounsaturated Fat	1.5 g	Copper	.039 mg
Polyunsaturated Fat	.578 g	Iron	.132 mg
Omega 3 Fatty Acid	.016 g	Magnesium	10.4 mg
Omega 6 Fatty Acid	.561 g	Manganese	.052 mg
Cholesterol	0 mg	Phosphorus	19.4 mg
Dietary Fiber	.353 g	Potassium	27.4 mg
Total Vitamin A	7.05 RE	Selenium	.171 mcg
A–Retinol	6.45 RE	Sodium	.378 mg
A–Carotenoi	.58 RE	Zinc	.115 mg
Thiamin–B1	.006 mg	Complex Carbohydrates	.116 g
Riboflavin–B2	.025 mg	Sugars	.207 g
Niacin–B3	.115 mg	Mono-Saccharide	0 g
Niacin Equivalent	.115 mg	Di-Saccharide	0 g
Vitamin B6	.004 mg	Alcohol	0 g
Vitamin B12	0 mcg	Caffeine	0 mg
Folate	1.4 mcg	Water	.328 g

☻ Sweet Fruit

Calories	18.4	Pantothenic	.031 mg
Protein	.338 g	Vitamin C	.278 mg
Carbohydrates	3.19 g	Vitamin D	0 mcg
Fat—Total	.661 g	Vitamin E-Alpha E	.062 mg
Saturated Fat	.129 g	Calcium	2.7 mg
Monounsaturated Fat	.385 g	Copper	.046 mg
Polyunsaturated Fat	.113 g	Iron	.177 mg
Omega 3 Fatty Acid	.003 g	Magnesium	5.18 mg
Omega 6 Fatty Acid	.11 g	Manganese	.022 mg
Cholesterol	0 mg	Phosphorus	10.2 mg
Dietary Fiber	.329 g	Potassium	40.1 mg
Total Vitamin A	8.57 RE	Selenium	.497 mcg
A–Retinol	0 RE	Sodium	.499 mg
A–Carotenoi	8.57 RE	Zinc	.097 mg
Thiamin–B1	.007 mg	Complex Carbohydrates	.309 g
Riboflavin–B2	.008 mg	Sugars	2.3 g
Niacin–B3	.085 mg	Mono-Saccharide	1.82 g
Niacin Equivalent	.085 mg	Di-Saccharide	.196 g
Vitamin B6	.014 mg	Alcohol	0 g
Vitamin B12	0 mcg	Caffeine	0 mg
Folate	1.21 mcg	Water	2.32 g

◎ Sweet Nuts

Calories	6.51	Pantothenic	.006 mg
Protein	.143 g	Vitamin C	.032 mg
Carbohydrates	.184 g	Vitamin D	0 mcg
Fat—Total	.619 g	Vitamin E-Alpha E	.026 mg
Saturated Fat	.056 g	Calcium	.941 mg
Monounsaturated Fat	.142 g	Copper	.014 mg
Polyunsaturated Fat	.391 g	Iron	.025 mg
Omega 3 Fatty Acid	.068 g	Magnesium	1.69 mg
Omega 6 Fatty Acid	.318 g	Manganese	.029 mg
Cholesterol	0 mg	Phosphorus	3.17 mg
Dietary Fiber	.045 g	Potassium	5.02 mg
Total Vitamin A	.124 RE	Selenium	.05 mcg
A–Retinol	0 RE	Sodium	.101 mg
A–Carotenoi	.124 RE	Zinc	.027 mg
Thiamin–B1	.004 mg	Complex Carbohydrates	.117 g
Riboflavin–B2	.001 mg	Sugars	.022 g
Niacin–B3	.01 mg	Mono-Saccharide	0 g
Niacin Equivalent	.01 mg	Di-Saccharide	.021 g
Vitamin B6	.006 mg	Alcohol	0 g
Vitamin B12	0 mcg	Caffeine	0 mg
Folate	.66 mcg	Water	.063 g

◎ Sweet Sesame

Calories	68	Pantothenic	.065 mg
Protein	2.39 g	Vitamin C	.185 mg
Carbohydrates	3.95 g	Vitamin D	0 mcg
Fat—Total	5.38 g	Vitamin E-Alpha E	.266 mg
Saturated Fat	.693 g	Calcium	13.5 mg
Monounsaturated Fat	1.84 g	Copper	.149 mg
Polyunsaturated Fat	2.6 g	Iron	.71 mg
Omega 3 Fatty Acid	.17 g	Magnesium	30.7 mg
Omega 6 Fatty Acid	2.42 g	Manganese	.177 mg
Cholesterol	0 mg	Phosphorus	68.1 mg
Dietary Fiber	.897 g	Potassium	67.9 mg
Total Vitamin A	.775 RE	Selenium	.943 mcg
A–Retinol	0 RE	Sodium	3.64 mg
A–Carotenoi	.775 RE	Zinc	.84 mg
Thiamin–B1	.067 mg	Complex Carbohydrates	.344 g
Riboflavin–B2	.013 mg	Sugars	2.85 g
Niacin–B3	.402 mg	Mono-Saccharide	2.36 g
Niacin Equivalent	.403 mg	Di-Saccharide	.042 g
Vitamin B6	.031 mg	Alcohol	0 g
Vitamin B12	0 mcg	Caffeine	0 mg
Folate	8.66 mcg	Water	.994 g

❂ Sweet Snack

Calories	60.2	Pantothenic	.057 mg
Protein	1.54 g	Vitamin C	.241 mg
Carbohydrates	5.78 g	Vitamin D	0 mcg
Fat—Total	3.81 g	Vitamin E-Alpha E	.25 mg
Saturated Fat	1.46 g	Calcium	28.6 mg
Monounsaturated Fat	.915 g	Copper	.055 mg
Polyunsaturated Fat	1.18 g	Iron	.208 mg
Omega 3 Fatty Acid	.137 g	Magnesium	9.61 mg
Omega 6 Fatty Acid	1.03 g	Manganese	.14 mg
Cholesterol	.302 mg	Phosphorus	18.3 mg
Dietary Fiber	.461 g	Potassium	52.4 mg
Total Vitamin A	.634 RE	Selenium	.441 mcg
A–Retinol	0 RE	Sodium	.728 mg
A–Carotenoi	.39 RE	Zinc	.153 mg
Thiamin–B1	.023 mg	Complex Carbohydrates	.657 g
Riboflavin–B2	.008 mg	Sugars	3.87 g
Niacin–B3	.38 mg	Mono-Saccharide	1.58 g
Niacin Equivalent	.38 mg	Di-Saccharide	.139 g
Vitamin B6	.027 mg	Alcohol	0 g
Vitamin B12	0 mcg	Caffeine	0 mg
Folate	5.15 mcg	Water	.549 g

❂ Trail Mix

Calories	30.6	Pantothenic	.039 mg
Protein	.876 g	Vitamin C	.074 mg
Carbohydrates	3.83 g	Vitamin D	0 mcg
Fat—Total	1.5 g	Vitamin E-Alpha E	.19 mg
Saturated Fat	.36 g	Calcium	9.66 mg
Monounsaturated Fat	.655 g	Copper	.025 mg
Polyunsaturated Fat	.384 g	Iron	.189 mg
Omega 3 Fatty Acid	.001 g	Magnesium	5.09 mg
Omega 6 Fatty Acid	.382 g	Manganese	.064 mg
Cholesterol	.07 mg	Phosphorus	11.8 mg
Dietary Fiber	.274 g	Potassium	42.7 mg
Total Vitamin A	.074 RE	Selenium	.495 mcg
A–Retinol	0 RE	Sodium	10.2 mg
A–Carotenoi	.018 RE	Zinc	.092 mg
Thiamin–B1	.022 mg	Complex Carbohydrates	1.26 g
Riboflavin–B2	.011 mg	Sugars	2.1 g
Niacin–B3	.402 mg	Mono-Saccharide	1.46 g
Niacin Equivalent	.402 mg	Di-Saccharide	.09 g
Vitamin B6	.012 mg	Alcohol	0 g
Vitamin B12	0 mcg	Caffeine	0 mg
Folate	3.81 mcg	Water	.441 g

☻ Truffles

Calories	57.2	Pantothenic	.023 mg
Protein	1.88 g	Vitamin C	0 mg
Carbohydrates	5.88 g	Vitamin D	0 mcg
Fat—Total	3.02 g	Vitamin E-Alpha E	.12 mg
Saturated Fat	2.06 g	Calcium	64.6 mg
Monounsaturated Fat	.401 g	Copper	.011 mg
Polyunsaturated Fat	.254 g	Iron	.128 mg
Omega 3 Fatty Acid	0 g	Magnesium	2.84 mg
Omega 6 Fatty Acid	.254 g	Manganese	.034 mg
Cholesterol	.806 mg	Phosphorus	5.81 mg
Dietary Fiber	.112 g	Potassium	10.7 mg
Total Vitamin A	.648 RE	Selenium	.12 mcg
A–Retinol	0 RE	Sodium	.097 mg
A–Carotenoi	0 RE	Zinc	.054 mg
Thiamin–B1	.007 mg	Complex Carbohydrates	.162 g
Riboflavin–B2	.002 mg	Sugars	3.54 g
Niacin–B3	.219 mg	Mono-Saccharide	.003 g
Niacin Equivalent	.219 mg	Di-Saccharide	.065 g
Vitamin B6	.004 mg	Alcohol	0 g
Vitamin B12	0 mcg	Caffeine	0 mg
Folate	2.36 mcg	Water	.025 g

☻ Vanilla Cake

Calories	47.8	Pantothenic	.042 mg
Protein	1.21 g	Vitamin C	.016 mg
Carbohydrates	5.15 g	Vitamin D	.377 mcg
Fat—Total	2.53 g	Vitamin E-Alpha E	.73 mg
Saturated Fat	.34 g	Calcium	7.24 mg
Monounsaturated Fat	1.24 g	Copper	.028 mg
Polyunsaturated Fat	.833 g	Iron	.518 mg
Omega 3 Fatty Acid	.016 g	Magnesium	7.56 mg
Omega 6 Fatty Acid	.816 g	Manganese	.086 mg
Cholesterol	0 mg	Phosphorus	16.9 mg
Dietary Fiber	.302 g	Potassium	26.4 mg
Total Vitamin A	35.2 RE	Selenium	.861 mcg
A–Retinol	32.2 RE	Sodium	17.2 mg
A–Carotenoi	2.9 RE	Zinc	.099 mg
Thiamin–B1	.058 mg	Complex Carbohydrates	4.59 g
Riboflavin–B2	.055 mg	Sugars	.262 g
Niacin–B3	.481 mg	Mono-Saccharide	.028 g
Niacin Equivalent	.482 mg	Di-Saccharide	.11 g
Vitamin B6	.005 mg	Alcohol	0 g
Vitamin B12	.007 mcg	Caffeine	0 mg
Folate	2.48 mcg	Water	5.24 g

⊚ Vanilla Drops

Calories	28.4	Pantothenic	.02 mg
Protein	.449 g	Vitamin C	.004 mg
Carbohydrates	3.2 g	Vitamin D	.403 mcg
Fat—Total	1.51 g	Vitamin E-Alpha E	.25 mg
Saturated Fat	.249 g	Calcium	1.3 mg
Monounsaturated Fat	.553 g	Copper	.006 mg
Polyunsaturated Fat	.633 g	Iron	.194 mg
Omega 3 Fatty Acid	.008 g	Magnesium	.976 mg
Omega 6 Fatty Acid	.627 g	Manganese	.028 mg
Cholesterol	0 mg	Phosphorus	5.02 mg
Dietary Fiber	.136 g	Potassium	5.42 mg
Total Vitamin A	37.6 RE	Selenium	1.41 mcg
A–Retinol	34.4 RE	Sodium	13.4 mg
A–Carotenoi	3.09 RE	Zinc	.029 mg
Thiamin–B1	.033 mg	Complex Carbohydrates	2.97 g
Riboflavin–B2	.021 mg	Sugars	.088 g
Niacin–B3	.247 mg	Mono-Saccharide	.038 g
Niacin Equivalent	.247 mg	Di-Saccharide	.017 g
Vitamin B6	.002 mg	Alcohol	0 g
Vitamin B12	.002 mcg	Caffeine	0 mg
Folate	1.11 mcg	Water	2.74 g

⊚ Vanilla Raisin Clusters

Calories	32.5	Pantothenic	.002 mg
Protein	.718 g	Vitamin C	.16 mg
Carbohydrates	5.91 g	Vitamin D	0 mcg
Fat—Total	.854 g	Vitamin E-Alpha E	.034 mg
Saturated Fat	.738 g	Calcium	26.3 mg
Monounsaturated Fat	.001 g	Copper	.015 mg
Polyunsaturated Fat	.007 g	Iron	.135 mg
Omega 3 Fatty Acid	.002 g	Magnesium	1.6 mg
Omega 6 Fatty Acid	.005 g	Manganese	.015 mg
Cholesterol	.302 mg	Phosphorus	4.7 mg
Dietary Fiber	.168 g	Potassium	36.3 mg
Total Vitamin A	.282 RE	Selenium	.322 mcg
A–Retinol	0 RE	Sodium	.581 mg
A–Carotenoi	.039 RE	Zinc	.013 mg
Thiamin–B1	.008 mg	Complex Carbohydrates	0 g
Riboflavin–B2	.004 mg	Sugars	4.94 g
Niacin–B3	.04 mg	Mono-Saccharide	3.14 g
Niacin Equivalent	.04 mg	Di-Saccharide	0 g
Vitamin B6	.012 mg	Alcohol	0 g
Vitamin B12	0 mcg	Caffeine	0 mg
Folate	.16 mcg	Water	.788 g

☺ Walnut Fudge

Calories	137	Pantothenic	.104 mg
Protein	3.72 g	Vitamin C	.43 mg
Carbohydrates	13.5 g	Vitamin D	.01 mcg
Fat—Total	7.97 g	Vitamin E-Alpha E	.192 mg
Saturated Fat	3.57 g	Calcium	119 mg
Monounsaturated Fat	1.15 g	Copper	.094 mg
Polyunsaturated Fat	2.63 g	Iron	.308 mg
Omega 3 Fatty Acid	.464 g	Magnesium	13.4 mg
Omega 6 Fatty Acid	2.14 g	Manganese	.194 mg
Cholesterol	3.94 mg	Phosphorus	42 mg
Dietary Fiber	.302 g	Potassium	64.1 mg
Total Vitamin A	8.44 RE	Selenium	.418 mcg
A–Retinol	6.03 RE	Sodium	11.2 mg
A–Carotenoi	1.49 RE	Zinc	.261 mg
Thiamin–B1	.033 mg	Complex Carbohydrates	.779 g
Riboflavin–B2	.044 mg	Sugars	9.51 g
Niacin–B3	.087 mg	Mono-Saccharide	0 g
Niacin Equivalent	.087 mg	Di-Saccharide	4.63 g
Vitamin B6	.041 mg	Alcohol	0 g
Vitamin B12	.037 mcg	Caffeine	0 mg
Folate	5.33 mcg	Water	2.57 g

☺ White Frosting

Calories	234	Pantothenic	.393 mg
Protein	35.5 g	Vitamin C	.532 mg
Carbohydrates	12.6 g	Vitamin D	.025 mcg
Fat—Total	.11 g	Vitamin E-Alpha E	.003 mg
Saturated Fat	.071 g	Calcium	123 mg
Monounsaturated Fat	.03 g	Copper	.009 mg
Polyunsaturated Fat	.003 g	Iron	.055 mg
Omega 3 Fatty Acid	.001 g	Magnesium	11.7 mg
Omega 6 Fatty Acid	.002 g	Manganese	.003 mg
Cholesterol	41 mg	Phosphorus	96.3 mg
Dietary Fiber	0 g	Potassium	156 mg
Total Vitamin A	638 RE	Selenium	2.16 mcg
A–Retinol	1.2 RE	Sodium	1406 mg
A–Carotenoi	.031 RE	Zinc	.595 mg
Thiamin–B1	.029 mg	Complex Carbohydrates	0 g
Riboflavin–B2	.599 mg	Sugars	4.7 g
Niacin–B3	.076 mg	Mono-Saccharide	0 g
Niacin Equivalent	.077 mg	Di-Saccharide	0 g
Vitamin B6	.032 mg	Alcohol	0 g
Vitamin B12	.375 mcg	Caffeine	0 mg
Folate	7.48 mcg	Water	52.2 g

⊚ Yummy Bananas

Calories	54.6	Pantothenic	.003 mg
Protein	1.63 g	Vitamin C	.082 mg
Carbohydrates	6.89 g	Vitamin D	0 mcg
Fat—Total	2.37 g	Vitamin E-Alpha E	.012 mg
Saturated Fat	2.07 g	Calcium	67.8 mg
Monounsaturated Fat	.002 g	Copper	.005 mg
Polyunsaturated Fat	.004 g	Iron	.11 mg
Omega 3 Fatty Acid	.001 g	Magnesium	1.27 mg
Omega 6 Fatty Acid	.002 g	Manganese	.007 mg
Cholesterol	.854 mg	Phosphorus	.871 mg
Dietary Fiber	.09 g	Potassium	17.5 mg
Total Vitamin A	1.05 RE	Selenium	.032 mcg
A–Retinol	0 RE	Sodium	.035 mg
A–Carotenoi	.359 RE	Zinc	.007 mg
Thiamin–B1	.002 mg	Complex Carbohydrates	.255 g
Riboflavin–B2	.003 mg	Sugars	4.36 g
Niacin–B3	.033 mg	Mono-Saccharide	0 g
Niacin Equivalent	.033 mg	Di-Saccharide	0 g
Vitamin B6	.006 mg	Alcohol	0 g
Vitamin B12	0 mcg	Caffeine	0 mg
Folate	.471 mcg	Water	.035 g

Index